INTRODUCTION

Dinner on the Ground. The words bring back pleasant memories of special days.

Who cannot recall carrying a gallon jar filled with homemade "sweet" tea? Or watching old men gather under a shade tree to wonder aloud about the events of the day? And can't we all remember wondering how long the preacher could go before a group of bored ladies left the service early to "prepare" the tables.

But the best memories were the mouth-watering bowls of food. Food so good and plentiful that a thin paper plate often collapsed under the weight.

Most people knew an unwritten requirement for attending a "dinner on the ground" was taking along your own secret recipe. Although there were no ribbons for first prize, everyone knew which foods made the top ten list.

In an effort to recapture many of these special dishes, we asked the senior adults who attend our annual Senior Adult Celebrations to submit their favorite recipe. This book is the result.

Here you will find old recipes and new ones. Some you may remember and some totally new. But all of them offer you something different for your next church or family gathering.

It is our wish that with these recipes you will find the same level of fun and fellowship that only comes at a "Dinner on the Ground."

Phil Waldrep
Phil Waldrep Ministries
Trinity, Alabama

COOKBOOK COMMITTEE

Phil Waldrep
Executive Editor

Tina Jones
Editor

Catherine Livingston
Typesetting

Ruth Bochte
Graphics

ACKNOWLEDGEMENTS

This cookbook is dedicated to all the group leaders who have attended a Senior Adult Celebration!

Dinner on the Ground

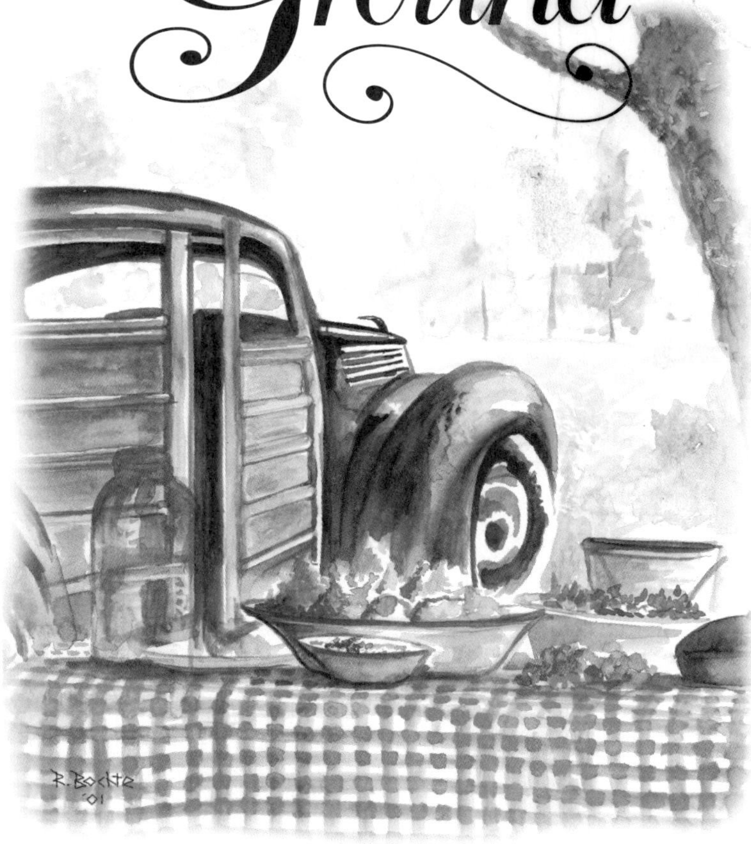

Official Cookbook of the Senior Adult Celebration!

PHIL WALDREP MINISTRIES
Trinity, AL

Phil Waldrep Ministries
P.O. Box 148
Trinity, Alabama 35673

First Printing November 2001
Second Printing December 2002

ISBN 0-9713746-0-0

WIMMER
COOKBOOKS
ConsolidatedGraphics
1-800-548-2537

TABLE OF CONTENTS

Phil Waldrep Ministries is a nonprofit organization committed to sharing the gospel by every means, traditional and non-traditional, and to provide quality resources for believers to grow in their relationships with God, their families and their friends. In addition to books and tapes, the ministry conducts major conferences, including:

Senior Adult Celebrations

Senior Adult Celebrations are events designed for retirees and senior adults. Held in major tourist areas, the Celebrations feature many of America's leading preachers, musicians, comedians and Christian celebrities. Among those who have appeared are Dr. David Jeremiah, Mark Lowry, George Beverly Shea, and Art Linkletter.

Women's Weekend Getaways

Women enjoy getting away with friends and focusing on their relationships with each other and the Lord. That is why the Women's Weekend Getaways are popular events for Christian women. The retreats begin on Friday night and conclude Sunday morning. They feature some of the most popular women speakers in the country.

Mountain Top Men's Retreat

Men from across the country gather each Spring for the Mountain Top Men's Retreat in Talladega, Alabama. The weekend event motivates men to develop their relationship with Christ, deepen their love for their family, and work more effectively in the local church.

Oasis Summer Student Camps and Student Celebrations

Phil Waldrep Ministries join hands with church youth ministers to provide a fun-filled spiritually enriching week for high school and college students each summer. Oasis camps feature special guests, exciting worship, Bible studies and messages designed for today's teen. In addition, the camps feature special activities that cause teens to grow closer to God, their friends, family and church. The Student Celebrations are designed to encourage and motivate students in their walk with God.

If you would like to know more about any of our exciting conferences, contact our office for a free brochure.

Phil Waldrep Ministries • (256) 355-1554

Celebrity Recipes

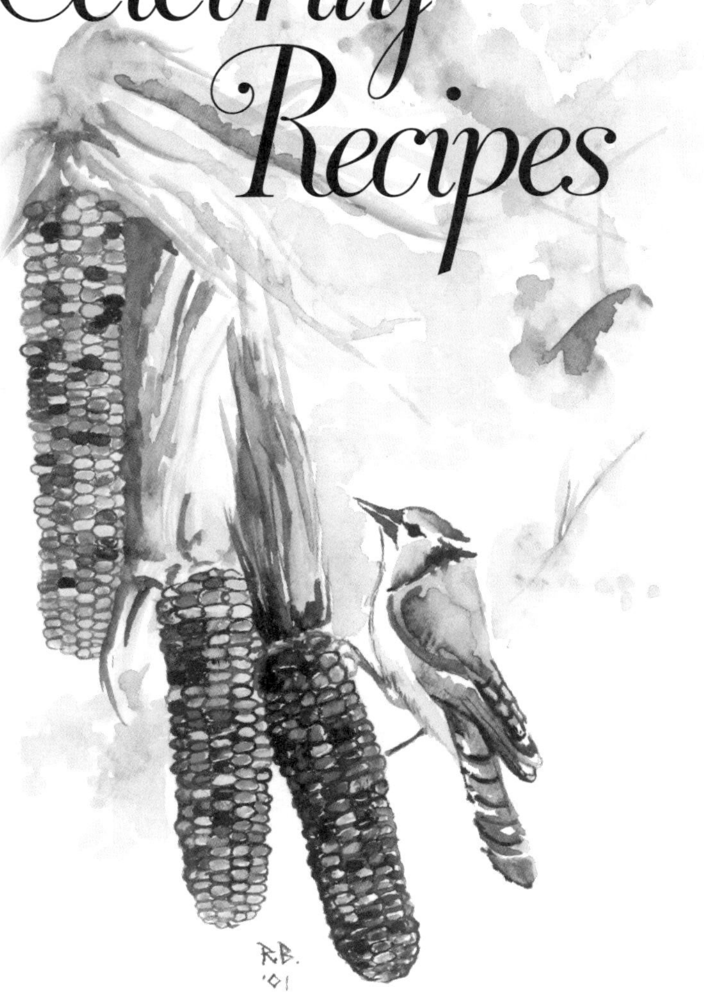

Through the Lord's mercies we are not consumed, because His compassions fail not. Lamentations 3:22

"The following personalities have, upon our request, provided their favorite recipes for your enjoyment."

TEXAS PECAN PIE

- 1½ cups Texas pecan halves
- 1 unbaked 9-inch pie shell
- 3 eggs
- 1 tablespoon butter, softened
- 1 cup dark corn syrup
- 1 tablespoon vanilla
- 1 cup sugar
- 1 tablespoon all-purpose flour

Arrange pecans in pie shell and set aside. Beat eggs until light. Add butter, corn syrup and vanilla. Stir until blended. Combine sugar and flour and blend into egg mixture. Pour into pie shell. Let stand until pecans rise to the surface. Bake at 350° for 45 minutes.

President George W. Bush

VIENNESE CRESCENT
(from "Chef Ariel")

- ¼ vanilla bean
- 1 cup powdered sugar
- 1 cup walnut meats
- 1 cup butter, room temperature
- ½ cup granulated sugar
- 2½ cups sifted all-purpose flour

Mince vanilla bean finely. Pound it in a mortar or pulverize it in a blender with 1 tablespoon powdered sugar. Mix with remaining powdered sugar. Cover, let stand preferably overnight. Reserve until ready to use. In a food processor, grind walnut meats into a paste. Transfer to a bowl; with wooden spoon, mix into a smooth dough with the butter, granulated sugar and flour. Shape dough about 1 teaspoon at time, into a small crescent. Bake on ungreased cookie sheets in a pre-heated 350° oven for 15 minutes or until lightly browned. Cool 1 minute and while still warm, roll cookies in prepared vanilla sugar.

Barbara Bush
Former First Lady of United States

RONALD REAGAN'S FAVORITE MACARONI AND CHEESE

½ pound macaroni
1 teaspoon butter
1 egg, beaten
1 teaspoon salt
1 teaspoon dry mustard
3 cups grated cheese, sharp
1 cup milk

Boil macaroni in water until tender and drain thoroughly. Stir in butter and egg. Mix mustard and salt with 1 tablespoon hot water and add to milk. Add cheese, leaving enough to sprinkle on top. Bake at 350° for about 45 minutes or until custard is set and top is crusty.

Nancy Reagan
Former First Lady of United States

NANCY REAGAN'S BROWNIES

3 squares semi-sweet baking chocolate
3 sticks butter
2 cups granulated sugar
1½ teaspoons salt
1 tablespoon vanilla
2 squares unsweetened baking chocolate
6 eggs
⅔ cup cake flour
1 teaspoon baking powder
2 cups finely chopped pecans
Powdered sugar

Melt chocolate and butter in top of double-boiler, then cool. Beat eggs and add sugar until light in color. Add chocolate mixture to egg mixture. Sift together flour, salt, and baking powder; add to other ingredients. Mix in vanilla and nuts. Pour into buttered and floured 12 x 18 inch pan. Bake in preheated 350° oven for 30 to 35 minutes. Cool, cut, then sprinkle with powdered sugar.

Nancy Reagan
Former First Lady of United States

TENNESSEE TREATS

2 cups dark brown sugar, firmly packed
2 whole eggs and 2 egg whites
2 tablespoons honey
1 teaspoon baking powder dissolved in ¼ cup boiling water
2 cups flour
½ teaspoon cinnamon
⅛ teaspoon allspice
⅛ teaspoon ground cloves
½ teaspoon salt
½ cup raisins
½ cup chopped dates
½ cup walnut pieces

Preheat over to 350°. In a large mixing bowl, mix brown sugar and eggs. Add honey and stir. Add baking powder to water and mix. Add water to mixing bowl. Combine flour and spices and stir into mixture. Add remaining ingredients and stir. Pour into greased 8 x 12 inch baking pan. Bake 350° for 30 to 40 minutes. To determine when treats are ready, insert toothpick. A nearly dry toothpick indicates they are done. Cut into squares while hot.

Tipper Gore
Wife of former Vice President Al Gore

MRS. MONDALE'S PUMPKIN BREAD

1½ cups sugar
1 teaspoon soda
¼ teaspoon baking powder
½ teaspoon cinnamon
½ teaspoon cloves
½ teaspoon nutmeg
¾ teaspoon salt
1⅔ cups flour
2 eggs
½ cup oil
1 cup canned pumpkin
½ cup water
½ cup chopped nuts
½ cup chopped dates

Sift together sugar, flour and all spices. Add eggs, oil, pumpkin and water and blend with beater. Add chopped nuts and dates. Bake at 350° for 1½ hours.

Joan Mondale
Wife of former Vice President Walter Mondale

WHITE CHILI

1 pound white beans
6 cups chicken broth
2 cloves minced garlic
2 medium chopped onions, divided
1 tablespoon oil
2 (4-ounce) cans of chopped green chiles
2 teaspoons ground cumin
1½ teaspoons dried oregano
¼ teaspoon ground cloves
¼ teaspoon cayenne pepper
4 cups diced chicken breast
3 cups grated Monterrey Jack cheese

Combine beans, chicken broth, garlic and ½ chopped onion. Simmer for 3 hours. Sauté remaining onion in oil. Add chiles, seasonings and mix thoroughly. Add to bean mixture. Add chicken breast and simmer for 1 hour.

8-10 servings

Bud Cramer
Alabama U. S. Representative

BAKED SQUASH

1½ pounds squash
1 medium onion, finely chopped
2 slices bread soaked in milk
1 egg
2-3 tablespoons butter
1 teaspoon salt
Dash pepper
1½ cups grated cheese

Cook squash until tender. Drain. Mash with butter, salt and pepper. Add slightly beaten egg, bread and onion finely chopped. Mix well. Pour half mixture in casserole and top with half of cheese. Add remaining mixture and top with remaining cheese. Bake at 350° for 30 minutes.

Albert P. Brewer
Former Governor of Alabama

HELEN HUNT'S SEASONING MIX

1 (26-ounce) box iodized salt
2 ounces paprika
3 ounces ground white pepper
3 ounces garlic powder
3 ounces onion powder
2 ounces chili powder
2 ounces Accent

Mix all ingredients together well and use as salt.

This is a mix I put together several years ago and I've shared it many times. When seasoning food: add until food tastes salty enough, then it is seasoned to perfection. Use generously on all foods unless recipe calls for other seasonings or spices in specific amounts. This is especially good for peas, butter beans, green beans, squash, steamed vegetables and cabbage. (I put it in canned green beans before they are pressured in canner.) I put the mix back into the 2 to 3-ounce containers to share with friends. It is a big amount of seasoning so have plenty of containers ready, pints jars, etc. All our family likes this.

Helen Hunt, Former First Lady of Alabama
(wife of Former Governor Guy Hunt)

SPINACH NOODLE DISH

1 cup grated Cheddar cheese
1 pound ground meat
6 ounces spinach noodles
1 (5-ounce) can tomato sauce
1 (5-ounce) can tomatoes
1 cup cottage cheese
Garlic or garlic salt to taste
1 green pepper, chopped
Mushrooms and sliced olives per taste

Fry meat; drain off fat. Cook noodles. Simmer tomatoes, tomato sauce, garlic, green pepper, mushrooms and olives about 10 minutes. Put in casserole in layers starting with noodles, then cottage cheese, sour cream and meat. Top with grated cheese. Cook in oven at 350° until it bubbles. Can be kept in refrigerator and reheated.

Lois and Art Linkletter

WILLARD SCOTT'S RECIPE FOR CHEESE GRITS SOUFFLÉ

Cook one (1) cup quick cooking grits in 4½ cups water with one (1) teaspoon salt. When done, stir in ¾ stick of butter and 1 stick Kraft's Garlic Cheese (optional on the garlic). Allow to cool.

Add two (2) beaten eggs into ¼ cup milk. Season with salt and pepper. Pour into buttered casserole dish and cover with 1 cup corn flakes (mix flakes with ¼ stick of butter). Cover well. Bake 40 to 45 minutes, 350°.

Delicious

Willard Scott

CHOLESTEROL-FREE MOLASSES COOKIES

- ½ cup milk
- ½ cup corn oil
- ¾ cup raisins
- 1 cup sugar
- 3 cups flour
- ½ cup molasses
- 1 teaspoon cinnamon
- ½ teaspoon nutmeg
- ½ teaspoon ground cloves
- 1 teaspoon soda
- ½ teaspoon salt
- ½ cup chopped walnuts

Preheat oven to 350°. Grease two baking sheets. Pour milk in small bowl, add raisins and allow to soak and soften. Measure remaining ingredients into large mixing bowl. Add milk and raisins and mix well. Drop generous spoonfuls onto baking sheet. Bake 12 to 15 minutes.

Dean Jones' Favorite Cookie Ever.

4 dozen

Dean Jones

HOT CARAMEL FRUIT

2 (29-ounce) cans Elberta Peaches
1 (16-ounce) can dark sweet cherries, pitted
1 (11-ounce) package dried apricots
Juice of ½ orange
Juice of ½ lemon
¼ teaspoon grated orange rind
¼ teaspoon grated lemon rind
1 cup firmly packed brown sugar
12 pitted dates
12 walnut halves

Preheat oven to 350°. Drain peaches and cherries (separately). Reserve peach juice. Turn fruit and peach juice into buttered baking dish. Add all ingredients except dates and walnuts. Bake, basting several times. While fruit bakes, stuff dates with walnut halves. About 15 minutes before fruit is done, arrange dates around the casserole, baste with syrup in bottom of baking dish and allow to finish baking. Bake 1½ to 2 hours.

Lory Jones,
Wife of Dean Jones

WHITE TOAST

Go to Kroger, Bi-Lo, K-Mart or Local Shell Station and buy 1 loaf of Wonder Bread and drive home observing speed limit. Go to kitchen, locate toaster, plug in toaster and adjust setting to medium. Insert bread into slots, press down button, watch bread go down. Wait patiently until toast pops up (if toaster is broken take out bread when you see smoke). Remove golden brown toast, go back to store, purchase butter, return home. Melt butter in microwave, take clean paint brush, brush melted butter on now cold toast. Eat slowly over waste basket so it can collect crumbs.

Doug Berkey
Humorist/Mime

STUFFED BURGER BUNDLES

1 package herb-seasoned stuffing mix
½ cup evaporated milk
1 pound ground beef
1 (10½-ounce) can condensed cream of mushroom soup
2 teaspoons Worcestershire sauce
1 tablespoon catsup

Prepare stuffing according to package directions. Combine evaporated milk and meat. Make 5 patties. On wax paper, pat each to 6-inch circle. Put ¼ cup stuffing in center of each; draw meat over stuffing and seal well. Place in 1½-quart casserole. Combine remaining ingredients and pour over meat. Bake uncovered at 350° for 45 minutes.

Ken Davis

REAL CORN BREAD

1 cup real cornmeal, ground from corn
1 tablespoon baking powder
¾ teaspoon salt
1 egg
Buttermilk
3 tablespoons canola or olive oil

Mix all ingredients together except oil and continue to add buttermilk until the mixture will pour with ease into the frying pan. Before pouring mixture into frying pan put the oil in frying pan and put it into the fire. When oil gets hot, pour oil into mixture and stir, then pour the whole mixture into the frying pan and make sure it is hot enough to sizzle when it is poured in. Then put frying pan into oven at 400° for about 15 to 20 minutes until it begins to separate from side of pan and slightly brown around edges. Put pan on top shelf of oven and turn oven to broil until cornbread browns on top. It is done now; take out and plop onto a plate.

It's great

Tom Lester

CHOCOLATE DELIGHT

½ cup Cocoa Puffs
½ cup Reese's Puffs
½ cup Cocoa Pebbles

Cover in ½% milk.

Dr. Charles V. Petty

SUGAR HIGH

½ cup Frosted Flakes
½ cup Lucky Charms
½ cup Cap'n Crunch

Cover in ½% milk.

Dr. Charles V. Petty

FRIENDLY CONVERSATION

1½ cups Rice Krispies

Cover in ½% milk; sit back and listen.

Dr. Charles V. Petty

BELLY BUSTER

Cereal and Popcorn!

Warning: Never mix three bran cereals in the same bowl.

Dr. Charles V. Petty

SPINACH SALAD

1 (10-ounce) package fresh baby spinach
⅔ cup sliced, toasted almonds
1 quart strawberries, sliced
¼ cup apple cider vinegar
½ cup sugar
1½ teaspoons finely chopped onion
¼ teaspoon paprika
¼ teaspoon Worcestershire sauce
½ cup vegetable oil

Wash spinach well and pull away any tough stems and discard. Put spinach in a large bowl. Combine vinegar, sugar, onion, paprika, Worcestershire sauce and vegetable oil in a cruet. Shake vigorously until the sugar dissolves. Serve over spinach. Put toasted almonds and sliced strawberries on salad. Toss, serve and enjoy!

Dennis Swanburg "The Swan"

CHICKEN VELVET SOUP

¾ cup soft butter
¾ cup flour
1 cup warm milk
1 pint hot chicken stock
1 cup warm cream
1 quart of chicken stock
1½ cups chopped, cooked chicken
¼ tablespoon salt
Pepper to taste

Simmer one 5-pound chicken (or 4-6 chicken breasts) in 2½ quarts water to prepare chicken stock. Blend butter and flour well. Add milk, 1 pint hot chicken stock, and 1 cup warm cream. Cook well then add 1 quart of chicken stock, chopped chicken, salt, and pepper. Do not boil but heat to the boiling point then keep warm until served.

This soup is a gourmet delicacy that is equally as beautiful to serve for special guests as it is nourishing for the family on a cold winter night. Better make a double batch!

Bill and Gloria Gaither

SUSIE'S RANCH STYLE BEANS

- 1 pound ground beef, browned and drained
- ½ medium onion, chopped
- 1 can stewed and chopped tomatoes
- 1 gallon can of "Ranch Style" beans

Mix all together, heat and enjoy!

Sprinkle grated cheese on top. Eat with cornbread or crackers.

Susie Luchsinger

PECAN STICKS

- ½ cup shortening (part butter)
- 2 cups brown sugar
- 2 eggs
- 1 cup chopped pecans
- 1 cup chopped dates (optional)
- 2 teaspoons vanilla
- ½ teaspoon salt
- 2 cups flour
- 2 teaspoons baking powder

Mix as butter cake, adding dates and nuts last. Spread rather thin on oiled jelly-roll pan (or one of that type). Bake in moderate oven for about 35 minutes.

Mother said she started making these for Daddy about 1920—before they were married.

Carolyn Newport,
Wife of Russell Newport

LEMON ICE BOX PIE

1 can Eagle Brand milk
1 carton Cool Whip
1 graham cracker crust
½ cup lemon juice

Mix Eagle Brand milk, Cool Whip and lemon juice. Put in crust and chill for 2 hours in refrigerator. Then serve.

Shae Billingsley
Wife of Charles Billingsley

PECAN PIE

1 cup sugar
2 tablespoons flour
2 eggs, slightly beaten
¾ cup light Karo
¼ cup cream or milk
1 teaspoon vanilla
1 cup broken pecans
1 tablespoon butter

Mix sugar and flour; add eggs, butter and beat. Add syrup, cream; mix well. Add vanilla; stir in pecans. Pour into unbaked pie shell and bake in moderate oven until set.

James W. Blackwood

OLD FASHIONED POTATO PONE

- 5 cups potatoes, ground
- 2 cups sugar
- ½ teaspoon allspice
- 1 teaspoon cinnamon
- ½ teaspoon cloves
- 4 eggs
- ⅔ cup self-rising cornmeal
- ¾ cup self-rising flour
- ¾ cup half-and-half or cream
- 1 stick margarine, melted

Grind potatoes with old fashioned meat grinder, grate or food processor. Mix potatoes, sugar, spices, flour and cornmeal. Then add melted butter, eggs and cream. Blend well and pour into a 9 x 13 inch pan or an old fashioned iron skillet greased with about 4 teaspoons butter or oil as you would cornbread. Bake at 350° until firm or about 30 minutes.

Price Harris

CRANBERRY WALNUT BREAD

- 2 cups apples, cored, peeled and chopped
- ¾ cup sugar
- 2 tablespoons oil
- 1 large egg
- 1½ cups all-purpose flour
- 1½ teaspoons baking powder
- ½ teaspoon baking soda
- 1 teaspoon cinnamon
- 1 cup cranberries, fresh or frozen
- ½ cup walnuts or pecans

Preheat oven to 350°. Grease and flour loaf pan. Combine apples, sugar and oil in mixing bowl. Add the egg and mix well. Combine dry ingredients in a separate bowl. Add to apple mixture. Stir in cranberries, apples and walnuts or pecans. Spread batter evenly into loaf pan. Bake one hour. Cake is done when toothpick inserted in cake is clean.

Great cake for Christmas

Addie Anderson,
Wife of Bill Anderson

CORN CHOWDER

3 cups fresh or frozen corn kernels
2 cups defatted broth (stock)
1 stalk celery (without leaves) finely chopped
1 medium onion, finely chopped
1 medium carrot, scraped and diced
1 potato, peeled and diced
1 red bell pepper, seeded and diced
4 cloves garlic, chopped
4 ounces Ortega green chiles, finely chopped
2 tablespoons rice vinegar
¼ teaspoon white pepper

Combine one half of the corn and 1 cup of stock in a blender until smooth. Pour into a large saucepan. Add remaining corn and stock, celery, onions, carrots, potatoes, bell peppers and garlic. Simmer 20 minutes. Add chiles, vinegar and pepper. Simmer 20 minutes more.

If you wanted it creamier, put about 2 cups back in blender and then add back to soup.

John Bisagno

CANDIED SWEET POTATOES

½ cup margarine
1 cup sugar
¾ cup water
3-4 large sweet potatoes, peeled and cut into 2-inch thick slices

Put water, sugar and margarine into skillet; let margarine melt and then add potatoes. Cover and simmer at 250° for 1 hour.

Ho[illegible] [illegible]e you've had a really good sweet, sweet potato with a

Junior Hill

BISCUITS FOR A "HAPPY" HUSBAND

2 cups self-rising flour
¼ cup Crisco
1 quart buttermilk (use enough to make dough batter)

Work Crisco into flour. Stir in buttermilk. Roll in flour bowl. Pinch off biscuits. Roll - Put in iron skillet (greased) pat tops with buttermilk. Bake 400°.

When John Ed and I married, Monteigne, who is John Ed's brother's wife, came over and brought all the above ingredients plus Mrs. Mary's (John Ed's mother) dough bowl. There was a note attached - "Please continue the Mathison tradition. John Ed always liked biscuits". Mrs. Mary had passed away a few months before and left these instructions with Monteigne for me. What a heritage and a blessing.

Lynn Mathison
Wife of John Ed Mathison

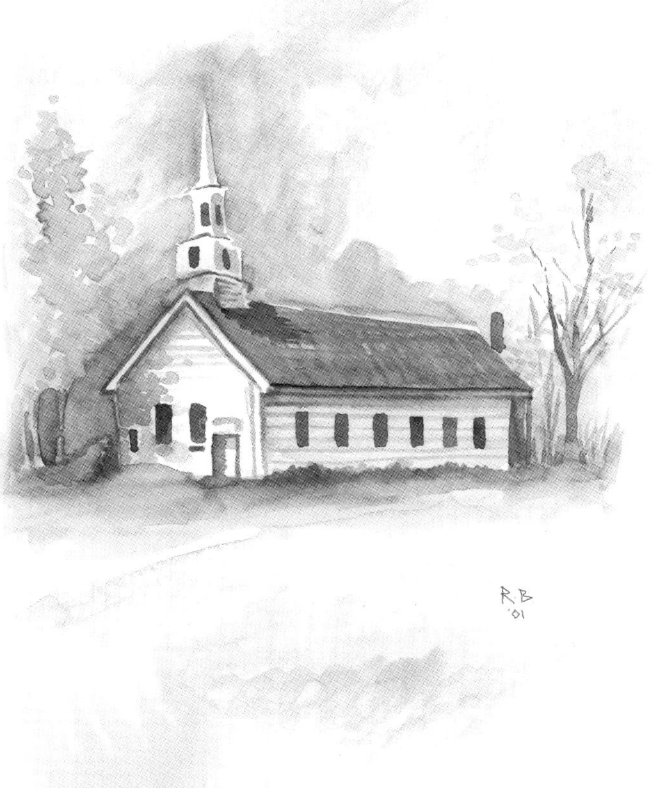

NORTH ALABAMA CHICKEN STEW

1 large chicken
1 onion (or 2 cups) chopped
7 medium potatoes, diced and cooked
3 medium potatoes, cooked and mashed
1 can cream of chicken soup
1 can cream of celery soup
1 (15-ounce) can cream corn
1 (15-ounce) can kernel corn
1½ cups dumpling macaroni
1 teaspoon red pepper
1 (46-ounce) can tomato juice
Salt and pepper to taste

Stew chicken with the onion for about 1 hour. As it cooks, peel, dice and cook potatoes. Crush the dumpling macaroni (I do this by putting it in a clean towel and breaking it with a hammer). When chicken is done, remove it from the water and debone it when cool. Add all ingredients to the chicken broth and cook on low for at least 2 hours. I recommend using a wire rack under you pan to keep the stew from scorching. Recipe makes about 10 quarts of stew. Freezes well.

This stew apparently has a North Alabama region origin as many of the Civic Organizations in that area cooks it in massive quantities and sells it by the gallon jugs on holidays. I have found very few people in the Memphis area who have ever heard of Chicken Stew, but all to whom I have served it seem to love it. Also, I grew up in Birmingham, Alabama, and no one there ever served it that I know of. Since the Lord moved us from Alabama 11 years ago, this dish is special to us as part of our home place as well as the memories of the many holidays we bought our gallon of Chicken Stew.

Sheryl Pitman (Mrs. Bob Pitman)

Appetizers

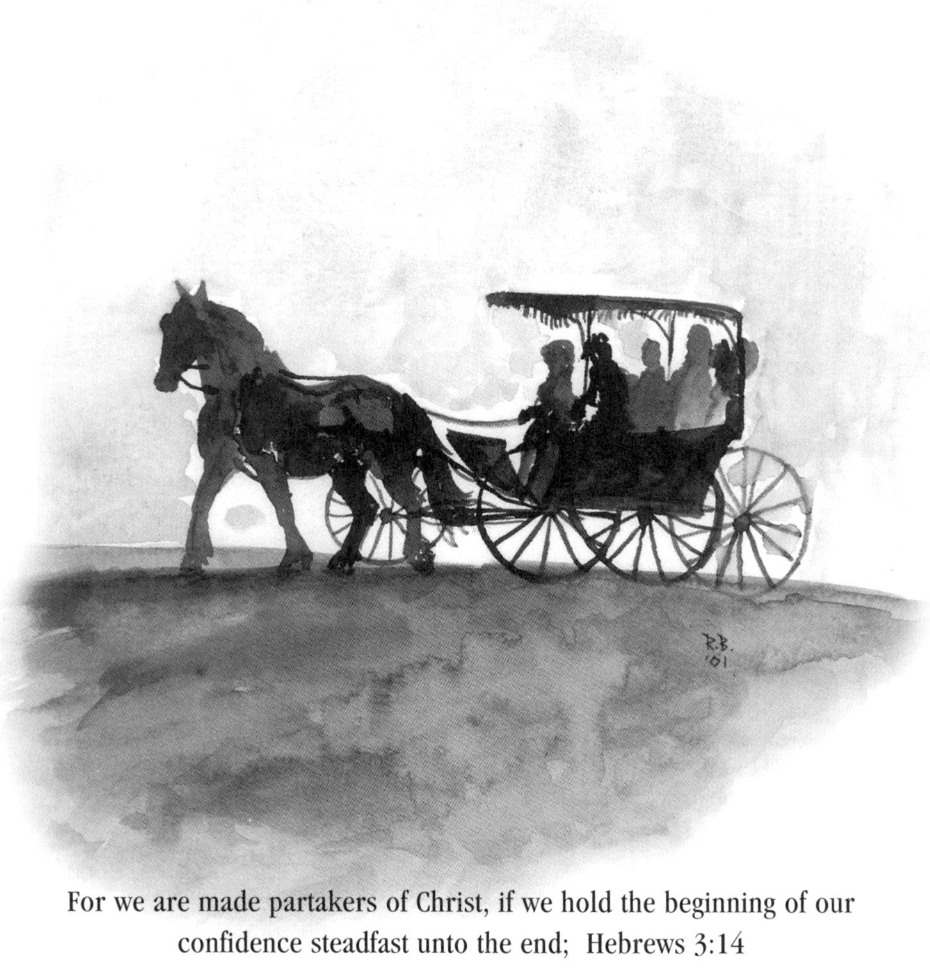

For we are made partakers of Christ, if we hold the beginning of our confidence steadfast unto the end; Hebrews 3:14

ZESTY SHRIMP DIP

- 2 (8-ounce) packages cream cheese
- 2 tablespoons mayonnaise
- 2 tablespoons milk
- 1 dash Worcestershire sauce
- ⅔ cup catsup
- 2 tablespoons minced onion
- 1 (4½-ounce) can shrimp

Mix well and chill overnight or for several hours.

Judy Field
Calvary Baptist Church
Dothan, AL

DIP FOR FRUIT

- 1 (8-ounce) package cream cheese
- 1 (7-ounce) jar marshmallow creme
- 2 drops orange flavoring
- ¼ teaspoon orange rind

Mix good and cool.

Shirley Morgan
Faith Baptist Church
Trinity, AL

DIP FOR APPLES

- 1 (8-ounce) package cream cheese, softened
- 1 teaspoon vanilla
- 3 large eating apples, sliced

Mix cream cheese and vanilla with mixer and serve with sliced apples.

Sara Lipham
Athens, AL

VIDALIA OR TEXAS SWEET ONION DIP

- 2-3 cups chopped onions
- 2 cups mayonnaise
- 2 cups shredded Swiss cheese
- 1 (8-ounce) can sliced water chestnuts, chopped

Mix all together and place in 350° oven until hot and bubbly. Serve with Frito's Scoop Chips.

Sharon Stringfellow
New Hope Baptist
Tuscaloosa, AL

HOT PIZZA DIP

- 1 (8-ounce) package cream cheese
- 1 teaspoon Italian seasoning
- 1 cup shredded mozzarella cheese
- ¾ cup shredded Parmesan cheese
- 1 (8-ounce) can pizza sauce
- 2 tablespoons chopped green peppers
- 2 tablespoons green onions, sliced

Combine cream cheese and Italian seasoning in 2-quart bowl; mix well. Combine cheeses; sprinkle half of cheese mixture over cream cheese. Spread pizza sauce over cheese; top with remaining cheese, pepper and onion. Microwave on HIGH 2 minutes; turn and microwave on HIGH 2 to 3 more minutes or until bubbly around edges.

Pizza dip may also be heated in conventional oven. Preheat oven to 350°. Bake 15 to 18 minutes or until cheese is melted and mixture is bubbling around edges.

12 servings—Serve with breadstick

Nancy Branham
Sawney's Creek Baptist
Ridgeway, SC

SOUTHWESTERN CHEESE DIP

1 pound American or Mexican cheese, cubed
1 (8-ounce) jar cheese spread
1 pound sliced bacon, cooked and crumbled
1 bunch green onions with tops, sliced
1 (4-ounce) can chopped green chiles
Raw vegetables or tortilla chips

Place cheeses in a 1½ qt microwave safe bowl. Top with bacon, onions and chiles. Microwave at 50% power for 6-8 minutes or until cheese is melted. Stirring every 2 minutes. Serve with vegetables or chips.

3 cups

Margaret Carroll
Alabaster, AL

WHITE FRUIT DIP

1 (8-ounce) package cream cheese
1 (8-ounce) jar marshmallow creme
1 tablespoon vanilla extract

With electric mixer, fluff the cream cheese. Add and mix marshmallow creme and vanilla. Chill if desired and serve with fruit.

Marguerite Nicholson
Russellville, AL

SPRING FEVER DIP

- 1 (11-ounce) can condensed chili beef soup
- 1 (3-ounce) package cream cheese, softened
- ½ cup sour cream
- 1 tablespoon water
- 1 teaspoon prepared mustard
- 1 teaspoon Worcestershire sauce
- ½ teaspoon chili sauce

In medium saucepan, heat soup and cream cheese, stirring constantly until cheese melts. Add remaining ingredients; mix well. Heat thoroughly and transfer to small crock pot. Serve warm with tortilla chips or corn chips.

Dorothy L. Kelly
First Baptist Church
Ozark, MO

GALA PECAN DIP

- 1 (8-ounce) package cream cheese
- 2 tablespoons milk
- 1 (8-ounce) package sliced beef, diced fine
- ¼ cup green pepper, chopped
- 2 tablespoons dehydrated onion flakes (can use fresh)
- ½ teaspoon garlic salt
- ¼ teaspoon black pepper
- ½ cup sour cream
- ½ cup chopped pecans
- 2 tablespoons butter
- ½ teaspoon salt

Combine cream cheese and milk; mix until well blended. Add beef, green peppers, onion, garlic salt and black pepper, mixing well. Fold in sour cream; spoon into baking dish. Heat pecans in melted butter and salt; sprinkle over cream cheese mixture. Bake at 350° for 20 minutes. Serve hot with crackers.

Rudy Branham
Sawney's Creek Baptist Church
Ridgeway, SC

ARTICHOKE CHEESE DIP

1 (14-ounce) can artichokes, chopped fine
1 cup Hellmann's light mayonnaise
¾ cup mozzarella or Monterrey Jack cheese, grated
1 cup Parmesan cheese
½ teaspoon garlic powder

Mix all ingredients well. Bake at 350° for 30 minutes or until bubbly. Serve with Wheat Thins or Nabisco Air Crisp Wheat Thins.

Carolyn Hartley
First Baptist Church
Palmerdale AL

SAUSAGE CHEESE BALLS

2 pounds uncooked sausage
1½ cups biscuit mix
4 cups shredded Cheddar cheese
½ cup finely chopped onions
½ cup finely chopped celery
½ teaspoon garlic powder

Mix all together and make 1-inch balls. Bake 15 minutes on ungreased cookie sheet at 375° preheated oven until golden brown. May be frozen uncooked.

For firmer texture, add an extra 3 cups biscuit mix and 2 cups cheese.

Minnie Gillam
Bronson, TX

CHILI BELLY

- 2 pounds ground beef
- 1 small onion
- 2 (15-ounce) cans ranch style beans
- 1 (10-ounce) can Ro-tel tomatoes and green chiles
- 2 (10¾-ounce) cans cream of mushroom soup

Brown chopped onion with the ground beef and drain. Mix all ingredients; put in crock pot and simmer 1½ to 2½ hours. Serve over Fritos.

Mary Lou Ellis
Alta Woods Baptist Church
Jackson, MS

HAM BALLS

- 2½ pounds ground ham
- 1½ pounds ground pork
- 1½ pounds ground beef
- 3 eggs
- 2 cups milk
- 3 cups crushed graham crackers
- 2 (10¾-ounce) cans tomato soup
- 1¾ cups brown sugar
- ¾ cup vinegar
- ½ teaspoon dry mustard

Mix ham, pork, beef, eggs, milk and crackers; make into balls and place in covered pan and bake for 45 minutes at 350°. Mix soup, brown sugar, vinegar and dry mustard in saucepan and simmer for a few minutes before pouring over meatballs. Pour sauce over meatballs and bake uncovered for 15 minutes.

Louise Grimme
Ozark, MO

PARTY HAM BALL

- 1 (8-ounce) package cream cheese
- 2 packages thin sliced ham, chopped
- 1 package green onions, chopped

Combine all together and roll in chopped pecans. Serve with crackers

Sidna Smalley
New Hope Church
Berry, AL

CHICKEN CHEESE BALL

- 3 (10-ounce) cans white chicken packed in water, drained
- 2 (8-ounce) packages no fat cream cheese
- 1 regular onion or 1 bunch green onions
- Lawry's seasoned salt
- Worcestershire sauce
- 1 cup finely chopped pecans

Mix all ingredients together seasoning to taste and roll in finely chopped pecans or just form into ball. Serve with any no fat or low fat crackers.

Lucy O'Donald
Burning Bush Baptist
Ringgold, GA

CHICKEN BALL

1 (12.5-ounce) can Swanson white chicken breast
1 (8-ounce) package non-fat cream cheese
1 stalk celery finely chopped
¼ teaspoon garlic powder
⅛ teaspoon onion salt
Pecans, coarsely chopped

Soften cream cheese and mix well with chicken. Add garlic powder and onion salt to taste. Stir in celery. Shape into ball and roll in pecans. Serve with crackers.

Serves approximately 8-10 people

Jeanette Statom
Westlawn Baptist Church
Huntsville, AL

TUNA BALL

1 (8-ounce) package cream cheese
1 (12-ounce) can tuna
¼ teaspoon chili powder
⅛ teaspoon onion slat
⅛ teaspoon curry powder

Combine cream cheese and tuna mixing well. Add seasonings and chill. Serve with crackers.

Fay M. Dinkin
Sawney's Creek Baptist Church
Ridgeway, SC

SWEET POTATO BALLS

2 cups mashed sweet potatoes
1 egg, beaten
2 tablespoons sugar
½ teaspoon salt
1 cup crispy rice cereal, crushed
1 package large marshmallows

Combine sweet potatoes and next 3 ingredients and form into balls around marshmallows. Roll in crushed cereal and bake at 375° about 20 minutes.

Lula Helms
Selma, AL

PINEAPPLE CHEESE BALL

2 (8-ounce) packages cream cheese
1 (8.5-ounce) can crushed pineapple, drained
⅓ cup chopped pecans
¼ cup green pepper, chopped
2 tablespoons chopped green onion
1 teaspoon seasoning salt

In a bowl combine cream cheese, pineapple, pecans, green pepper, green onion and salt. Mix thoroughly and shape into a ball and roll in remaining chopped pecans. Cover and chill several hours or overnight. Serve with assorted crackers.

Jeanette Statom
Westlawn Baptist Church
Huntsville, AL

SALMON APPETIZERS

1 (15-ounce) can salmon
1 (8-ounce) package cream cheese
4 tablespoons mild salsa
2 tablespoons chopped fresh parsley
1 teaspoon cumin (optional)
8 flour tortillas (8-inch)
1 teaspoon dried cilantro

Drain salmon; remove bones. Combine salmon, cream cheese, salsa, parsley, cilantro and cumin. Mix well and spread about 2 tablespoons of mixture over each tortilla. Roll up lightly and wrap individually with plastic wrap. Refrigerate 2 to 3 hours. Slice into bite-size pieces.

48 servings

Betty Denning
Algier, NC

PARTY SANDWICH FILLING

1 (8-ounce) package cream cheese
¾ cup chopped pecans
¼ cup chopped bell pepper
¼ cup chopped onion
3 tablespoons pimento
1 tablespoon catsup
3 hard-boiled eggs
¾ teaspoon salt
⅛ teaspoon black pepper

Mix all ingredients well and spread between bread slices.

Annie Ruth Austin
Tabernacle Baptist Church
Union, SC

CHEESE STRAWS

- 1 pound New York State extra sharp cheese, grated
- 4 sticks corn oil margarine
- 4½ cups plain flour
- 1¾ teaspoons cayenne pepper
- ½ teaspoon salt
- 2 cups finely chopped pecans

Cream cheese and margarine together. Add flour, pepper and salt and blend well. Add nuts. Squeeze through a cookie press onto an ungreased cookie sheet. Bake at 350° for 12 to 15 minutes

These freeze beautifully—if they stay around that long.

16-18 dozen

Mozelle Buff Wilson
Calvary Baptist Church
Morganton, NC

PARTY CHEESE WREATH

- 1 (8-ounce) package sharp Cheddar cheese, shredded
- 2 (8-ounce) packages cream cheese
- 1 teaspoon lemon juice
- 1 tablespoon red bell pepper, finely chopped
- 1 tablespoon green pepper, finely chopped
- 2 teaspoons Worcestershire sauce
- Dash ground red pepper

Beat Cheddar cheese and cream cheese with mixer on medium speed until well blended. Add lemon juice, bell pepper, onion, Worcestershire sauce and ground red pepper and mix well. Refrigerate several hours or overnight. Place drinking glass in center of serving patter. Drop round tablespoons of mixture to form ring around glass, just touching outer edge of glass; smooth with spatula. Remove glass. Garnish with fresh parsley and red pepper stars. Serve with crackers.

2 cups

Dean Smith
Derma Baptist Church
Calhoun City, MS

PINEAPPLE CHEESE LOG

- 2 (8-ounce) packages cream cheese
- 1 (3½-ounce) can crushed pineapple, drained
- 2 cups pecans, chopped very fine
- ¼ cup chopped bell pepper
- 1 tablespoon seasoned salt

Beat cream cheese until smooth. Add pineapple, 1 cup pecans, green pepper and salt. Shape into 2 logs. Roll into remaining nuts. Wrap in foil and chill over night.

Lois Morris
Crosspointe Baptist Church
Owensboro, KY

HAM N' CHEESE PUFFS

- 1 stick butter
- 1½ cups shredded Cheddar cheese
- ¼ cup finely chopped baked ham
- ¼ teaspoon Worcestershire sauce
- 1 cup sifted all-purpose flour
- Dash cayenne pepper

In mixing bowl, combine butter, cheese, ham and seasonings. Blend in flour. Shape dough into a smooth ball. Roll into balls the size of large marbles and place on baking sheet. Bake in 350° oven 15 to 18 minutes. Serve piping hot.

Freezes well unbaked

36 balls

Jean Hood
Santa Fe Baptist Church
Santa Fe, TN

MAURICE'S CHEESE ROLL

1 (16-ounce) package cream cheese
1 cup pecans, ground
1 teaspoon A-1 sauce
1 garlic clove
Chili powder, to taste

Set out cream cheese until room temperature. Chop pecans very fine and grate or grind garlic clove very fine. Beat cream cheese with mixer until smooth. Add pecans, A-1 sauce and grated garlic. Beat until all ingredients are blended together. Form mixture into a roll, wrap in waxed paper and chill. Sprinkle with chili powder. Set out one hour before serving.

Willene Holton
First Baptist Church
Alma, GA

HAM AND CHEESE TARTS

1 can Big Country Biscuits
1 package deli ham
1 cup Cheddar cheese
Butter and garlic, if desired

Press each biscuit into a 5-inch round. Fill with one tablespoon each of chopped deli ham and cheese. Fold. Seal edges with a fork. Bake at 400° for 10 to 15 minutes.

Jeanette Statom
Westlawn Baptist Church
Huntsville, AL

BACON WRAPPED PECANS

1 pound good bacon
1 pound pecan halves

Set bacon out of refrigerator for about 1 hour before using. Cut each bacon strip into 3 equal parts. Place 2 pecan halves together and wrap bacon around pecans. Place seam side down on microwave bacon pan. Cover with paper towel. Microwave 20 to 25 pieces for 5 to 6 minutes or until done.

May be stored in refrigerator for up to 10 days or frozen and used later. You may want to sauté pecans in butter and garlic before wrapping in bacon to give a little different taste.

50-60

Carolyn Hartley
FBC, Palmerdale, AL

TEXAS CAVIAR

1 (14¾-ounce) can yellow whole kernel corn, drained
1 (11-ounce) can white shoepeg corn, drained
1 (15-ounce) can pinto beans, drained
2 (15-ounce) cans black-eyed peas, drained
2 cups diced bell pepper
1 cup chopped green onions
½ cup chopped jalapeño pepper
1 tablespoon garlic salt
1 (16-ounce) bottle Italian dressing
1 (16-ounce) can pitted black olives, sliced
Black pepper to taste

Mix all ingredients the night before serving. Refrigerate. Serve with corn chips or bite size Tostitos.

Keeps for several weeks in refrigerator

Myrtle Campbell
Calvary Baptist Church
Dothan, AL

CAVIAR

1 (15-ounce) can black-eyed peas, drained
¼ cup cider vinegar
¼ cup cooking oil
1 small onion, chopped
Tabasco, to taste

Mix oil, vinegar and Tabasco. Pour over peas and onions. Marinate at least 8 hours. Serve with toasted round or thin wheat crackers.

Shirley Whitehead
Highland Baptist Church
Vicksburg, MS

HOT SPICY MILK DRINK

2 cups water
¼ cup whole cloves
½ cup red cinnamon candies
½ cup sugar
Milk

Mix together in saucepan and simmer 15 minutes, stirring occasionally. Strain. Use 2 tablespoons per cup of milk. Serve in hot mugs, topped with marshmallows.

8 servings

Yvonne Sherrill
Mt. Hebron Baptist Church
Spruce Pine, AL

PEPPERMINT COCOA

3 (4½-inch) peppermint sticks
1 cup powdered sugar
1 cup powdered non-dairy creamer
¾ cup unsweetened cocoa

Place peppermint sticks in an airtight bag; beat to a powder with a mallet. Combine peppermint with sugar, creamer and cocoa. Add ½ teaspoon to ¾ cup boiling water for each serving. Store remaining in a jar or airtight bag.

8 servings

Wanda Jones
Montevallo, AL

CAPPUCCINO MIX

1 cup non-dairy creamer
1 cup chocolate milk mix
⅔ cup instant coffee granules
½ cup sugar
½ teaspoon ground cinnamon
¼ teaspoon ground nutmeg

Combine ingredients and mix well. Store in tight container. Use 4 teaspoons per cup of boiling water.

33 servings

Bobbie Hill
Pleasant Grove Baptist Church
Coatfield, TN

BAPTIST PUNCH

2 packages Kool Aid
2 cups sugar
1 (46-ounce) can pineapple juice
1 (32-ounce) bottle ginger ale

Mix and add water to make jug about ¾ full. Put in freezer. Shake jug about once an hour to slush. When read to serve add ginger ale.

B
Harmony Fr

SLUSH FRUIT PUNCH

- 1 cup sugar
- 1½ cups water
- 1 (46-ounce) can pineapple juice
- 1 (32-ounce) can cranapple juice
- 1 (12-ounce) can frozen lemonade, thawed
- 1 (32-ounce) bottle ginger ale

Mix sugar and water over low heat until mixed well and cool. Mix juices together well and then mix with sugar and water mixture and freeze. (May be made a week before using.) Take out of freezer 2 to 3 hours before serving. Put slush in punch bowl. Add ginger ale to the slush in punch bowl. Serve.

Serves 20-25 people in 4-ounce cups

Eleanor Kay
Whitesburg Baptist Church
Huntsville, AL

ORANGE JUICE, JULIUS

- 1 (6-ounce) can frozen orange juice
- 1 cup milk
- 1 cup water
- ½ cup sugar
- ½ teaspoon. vanilla
- 10-12 ice cubes

Blend in blender until ice is crushed.

Violet Justice
Oliver Springs, TN

STRAWBERRY PUNCH

2 (0.15-ounce) packs of strawberry Kool-Aid, unsweetened
1 (46-ounce) can pineapple juice
1 (6-ounce) can frozen orange juice
2 cups sugar
½ gallon raspberry sherbet

Mix Kool-Aid, pineapple, orange juice and sugar together and add enough water to make a gallon. Add sherbet to gallon of juice mixture.

Brenda Whisenant
East Booneville Baptist Church
Booneville,MS

HOT SPICED TEA

1 cup orange Tang
2 cups sugar
½ cup instant tea
1 (0.15-ounce) package lemonade mix
1 teaspoon cloves
1 teaspoon cinnamon

Mix all ingredients. Store in a covered container. Use 2½ teaspoons to one cup of hot water.

Lula Helms
Selma, AL

INSTANT RUSSIAN TEA

2 (0.15-ounce) packages dry lemonade
2½ cups sugar
½ cup instant tea
2 cups dry Tang
1 teaspoon ground cinnamon
2 teaspoon ground cloves

Mix together. Add 2 teaspoons for each cup of hot water.

Ginny Brooke
Parkwood Baptist Church
Concord, NC

COOL FRUIT SMOOTHIE

1 (21-ounce) can fruit filling (any flavor)
½ cup non-fat plain yogurt
1 medium banana
3 cups ice
Mint leaves (optional)

In blender, combine all ingredients (except mint) and blend until smooth, stopping to scrape sides of blender as necessary. Pour into glass and garnish with sprig of mint, if desired.

4 servings

Gail Doe
Westwood Baptist
Alabaster, AL

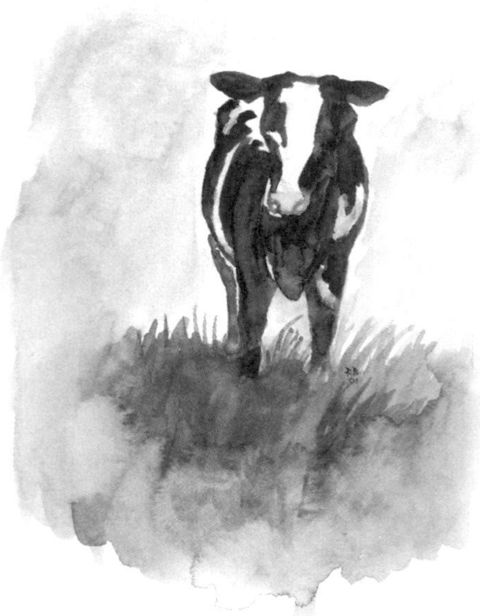

Breads

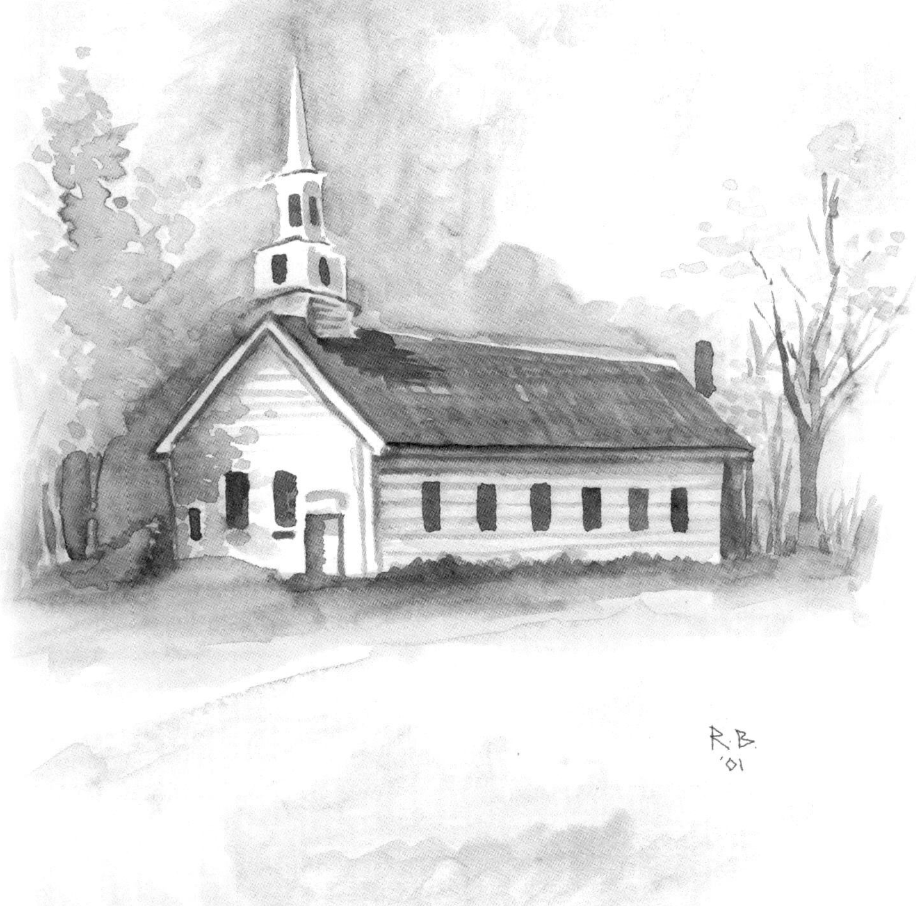

Man doth not live by bread only, but by every word that proceedeth out of the mouth of the Lord doth man live. Deuteronomy 8:3

SWEET "TATER" BISCUITS

- ¾ cup cooked sweet potatoes, mashed
- ⅔ cup milk
- 3 tablespoons melted butter
- 1¼ cups plain flour
- 4 teaspoons baking powder
- ½ teaspoon salt

Mix mashed potatoes, milk, and melted butter. Sift dry ingredients together; add to potato mixture to make a soft dough. Turn out on a floured board and toss lightly until outside looks smooth. Roll out ½-inch thick; cut with floured biscuit cutter. Bake on greased pan at 450° for about 14 minutes.

1 dozen biscuits

Marguerite Dinkins
Sawney's Creek Baptist Church
Ridgeway, SC

CHEDDAR GARLIC BISCUITS

- 2 cups biscuit baking mix
- ⅔ cup milk
- ½ cup shredded Cheddar
- 2 tablespoons melted butter
- ⅛ teaspoon garlic powder

Heat oven to 450°. Mix biscuit mix, milk and cheese to form soft dough. Drop by spoonfuls onto ungreased cookie sheet. Bake 8 to 10 minutes. Mix butter and garlic powder and brush over warm biscuits.

Ginny Brooks
Parkwood Baptist Church
Concord, NC

CHEESE BISCUITS

1 pound sharp Cheddar, grated
1 pound butter, softened
4-5 cups plain flour
2 teaspoons baking powder
2 cups pecan halves
Dash Tabasco sauce

Blend grated cheese and softened butter. Add flour, baking powder and Tabasco sauce. Roll into small balls, place on cookie sheet and press a pecan half in center of each ball to flatten. Bake 10 to 15 minutes in 325° oven. Watch carefully. Biscuits need to be crisp. Do not let pecans over brown.

Irene Wilson
Harlan Baptist Church
Harlan, KY

BREAKFAST MUFFINS

1 pound sausage, browned
1 (10¾-ounce) can Cheddar cheese soup
3½ cups biscuit baking mix
Small amount of water

Combine sausage, soup and biscuit mix. Add water until consistency is a little thicker than cake mix. Put in muffin tins. Bake at 350° until light brown.

Patty Woodham
New Hope Baptist
Fayette, AL

SWEET POTATO ROLLS

1 can Hungry Jack biscuits
2-3 sweet potatoes
2 cups water
2 cups sugar
1 teaspoon vanilla
1½ sticks margarine

Separate biscuits into 20 pieces, roll out and sprinkle with nutmeg. Cut potatoes into finger size strips. Place 2 potato strips in each biscuit piece and roll up. Melt margarine in 9 x 13 inch baking dish. Place biscuits in dish seam-side down. Makes 2 rows. Heat water, sugar and vanilla until sugar dissolves and pour over rolls. Bake at 350° for 30 minutes.

Gertie Key
Fellowship Baptist Church
Mt. Airy, NC

CHOCOLATE ROLLS

Bisquick mix
1 cup sugar
4 tablespoons cocoa
1 teaspoon vanilla
2 cups milk

Mix Bisquick dough as directed for batch of biscuits. Roll out in a rectangular shape. Mix sugar and cocoa and sprinkle over dough. Roll up and cut in 2-inch wide rolls. Place in 9 x 13 inch baking dish. Mix vanilla and milk and pour over rolls. Bake in 350-400° oven for 30 to 40 minutes.

Mary Harris
Cornerstone Baptist Church
Hartwell, GA

BROCCOLI BREAD

- 1 (8½-ounce) Jiffy corn muffin mix
- 1 (10-ounce) package chopped broccoli, thawed and drained
- 1 small onion, chopped
- 1 stick butter, melted
- 4 eggs, slightly beaten
- 1 teaspoon salt
- 1 (8-ounce) carton small curd cottage cheese

Mix all ingredients in bowl, adding Jiffy mix last. Bake in greased 9 x 13 inch baking dish at 400° for 25 minutes.

Violet Justice
Oliver Springs, TN

SALMON HUSH PUPPIES

- 1 (14¾-ounce) can salmon, reserve ¼ cup liquid
- ½ cup flour
- ½ teaspoon soda

Mix salmon, flour and soda along with reserved liquid together. Shape into balls and deep fry.

Sue Gargis
Leighton, AL

HAMBURGER ROLLS

- 1 (8-ounce) can crescent rolls
- 1 (1¼-ounce) envelope onion soup mix
- 1 pound hamburger
- 2-3 cups grated sharp cheese

Brown hamburger and drain. Add other ingredients except rolls. Cut rolls in half. Put small amount of mixture on roll. Fold over from each side, then fold up from bottom. Bake at 375° for about 15 minutes.

Lynn Satterfield
Central Baptist
Cowpens, SC

BREADS

LUEBERRY MUFFINS

1 egg
½ cup sugar
1 cup blueberries

...gredients except berries, then fold in the berries lightly. Put in greased muffin pans and bake at 400° for 20 to 30 minutes.

1 dozen

Julia Corn
Lake Wateree Baptist Church
Ridgeway, SC

STRAWBERRY BREAD

3 cups flour
1 teaspoon soda
1 teaspoon salt
1 teaspoon cinnamon
2 cups sugar
1¼ cups oil
4 eggs well beaten
2 cups frozen strawberries, including juice

Mix all ingredients together by hand. Bake in 2 loaf pans at 350° for 1 hour until done.

Delicious warm with butter

Grace Akin
Westlawn Baptist Church
Huntsville, AL

STRAWBERRY NUT BREAD

3 cups flour
1 teaspoon baking soda
1 teaspoon salt
1 tablespoon cinnamon
2 cups sugar
4 eggs, beaten
1¼ cups vegetable oil
1¼ cups chopped nuts
2 cups sliced strawberries, thawed

Combine dry ingredients. Add eggs, oil, strawberries, and pecans. Stir just enough until all the ingredients are moistened. Spoon batter into well greased loaf pan or 1 Bundt pan. Bake at 350° for 60 or 70 minutes or until bread tests done. Cool in pans for 5 minutes. Remove to wire rack to cool.

Line pan with wax paper and grease all around to speed cleanup.

Sue McCrory
Calvary Baptist Church
Dothan, AL

APPLESAUCE MUFFINS

2 sticks margarine
2 cups sugar
2 eggs
1 teaspoon vanilla
4 cups plain four
3 teaspoons cinnamon
1 teaspoon cloves
2 teaspoons allspice
1 (16-ounce) can applesauce
3 teaspoons soda
1 cup nuts or raisins (optional)

Add applesauce and soda in large bowl. This will begin to bubble. Cream margarine and sugar. Add eggs one a time and beat well. Add vanilla. Sift together the flour and spices. Add to margarine and sugar mix. Add applesauce and soda mixture. Pour into greased muffin tins. Cook in 400° oven for approximately 10 minutes.

Do not have to cook all at one time. Use what you want and store balance in tight container in refrigerator until ready to bake more muffins. When you have some made ahead, this makes for a quick breakfast or dessert.

Bobby Sue Green
Trinity Baptist Church
Childersburg, AL

MAYONNAISE ROLLS

1 [illegible]f-rising flour
½ c[illegible]ilk
2 tablespoons mayonnaise
Pinch sugar

Mix well with spoon and put in muffin pans. Bake 20 minutes at 450°.

Opal Ferguson
Enon Baptist Church
Danville, AL

GOLDEN CROWNS

2 packages dry yeast
½ cup warm water
½ cup milk
½ cup sugar
¼ cup salad oil
1 teaspoon salt
2 eggs
4½ cups sifted flour
1½ sticks butter
1½ cups sugar
2 tablespoons cinnamon
1 cup chopped nuts

Add yeast to warm water to soften. Scald milk; add ½ cup sugar, oil, and salt. Mix well and combine with yeast. Add eggs and stir in flour. Knead on floured board until smooth and elastic. Place in greased bowl and cover with damp cloth. Let rise until double in bulk, about 2 hours. Punch down, and punch down. Let rest 10 minutes while preparing butter and nut topping. Melt butter; combine sugar, cinnamon and nuts. Pinch off small pieces of dough with buttered hands, shape into balls—size of golf balls. Roll each ball in melted butter and then in sugar-nut mixture. Arrange in well-greased 9-inch tube pan. Sprinkle on remaining sugar-nut topping. Cover and let rise until doubled, about 2 hours. Bake in 375° oven for 40 minutes. Break nuggets apart to serve.

Norene Morris
Wayside Baptist Church
Miami, FL

NEVER FAIL DINNER ROLLS

- 2 cups water, divided
- ½ cup margarine
- ½ cup Crisco
- ¾ cup sugar
- 1½ teaspoons salt
- 2 packages yeast
- 2 eggs
- 6 cups bread flour

Put 1 cup water in medium saucepan, bring to boil and remove from heat. Add shortening and margarine; stir until melted. Add sugar and salt; let cool to lukewarm and add eggs. Set aside. In large mixing bowl put 1 cup warm water and sprinkle yeast over water (don't have water too hot, it will kill the yeast). Stir until yeast is dissolved. Add the first mixture to water and yeast; stir in flour. Cover and put in refrigerator overnight. Remove next day. Let set for 1 hour. Roll out to desired thickness and cut with biscuit cutter. Place on greased cookie sheet. Brush with butter; let stand 2 hours. Bake at 400° for 12 to 18 minutes.

Ruth Jones
Community Baptist Church
Elkmont, AL

MEXICAN CORN BREAD

- 1½ cups self-rising white cornmeal
- 2 eggs
- ½ teaspoon salt
- 1 teaspoon baking powder
- ⅓ cup vegetable oil
- 1 pod chili pepper or ½ teaspoon Cayenne pepper
- 1 (8¾-ounce) can cream style corn
- 1 cup grated Cheddar cheese
- 1 cup buttermilk

Mix all ingredients. Pour in well greased iron skillet. Bake at 350° for 45 to 50 minutes.

Nancy W. Cheek
Brookwood Baptist Church
Haw River, NC

BLACK-EYED PEA CORNBREAD

- 1 pound hot sausage
- 1 onion
- 1 (16-ounce) box cornbread mix
- 1 cup chopped green pepper
- 1 (14¾-ounce) can cream corn
- 1 (15½-ounce) can black-eyed peas
- 2 eggs
- 1 cup buttermilk
- ⅓ cup vegetable oil

Cook sausage and onion together until brown. Drain and set aside. Combine cornbread mix with dry ingredients. Beat eggs, buttermilk and oil together. Add to dry ingredients. Add sausage and onion. Spray pan with nonstick cooking spray and fill pan. Bake in preheated 325° oven for 45 to 50 minutes.

Evelyn Cooper
Providence Baptist Church
Keithville, LA

SOUTHERN HUSH PUPPIES

- ½ cup self-rising cornmeal
- ½ cup self-rising flour
- 1 egg
- 1 finely chopped medium onion
- Milk or buttermilk

Mix all ingredients thoroughly and moisten with milk or buttermilk just enough to slide off spoon into boiling oil in which fish has been fried. Cook until they float and are golden brown.

Ruby Bentley
Lincolnton Baptist Church
Lincolnton, GA

Soups & Salads

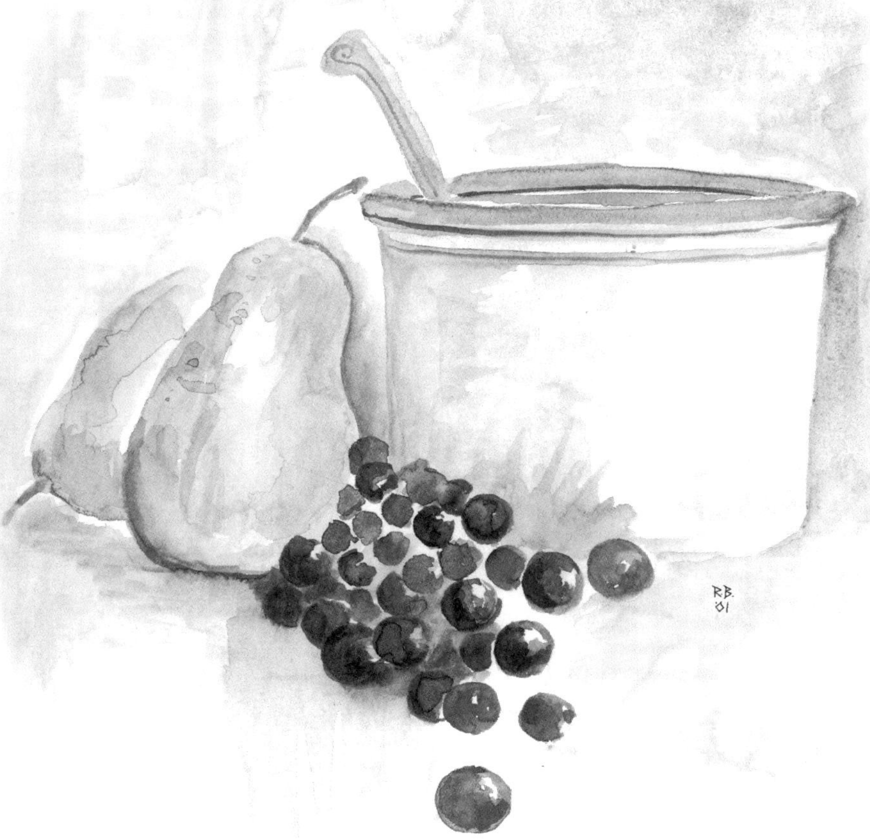

Let your conversation be always full of grace, seasoned with salt, so that you may know how to answer everyone. Colossians 4:6

WHITE CHILI

5 (15.8-ounce) cans great Northern beans
1 (10-ounce) can chicken
1 (4½-ounce) can chopped green chiles
1 small onion, chopped
2 tablespoons ground cumin
2 teaspoons white pepper
2 tablespoons chopped parsley
2 (16-ounce) cans chicken broth
8 ounces Pepper Jack cheese
Water to cover beans

Mix all ingredients, (except cheese). Add enough water with chicken broth to cover beans. Cover let simmer about 30 minutes. Add cheese to your liking.

8-10 servings

Faye Webster
Glencoe, KY

CHILI

3 pounds hamburger meat
3 cups water
1 tablespoon chili powder
1 tablespoon salt
1¼ teaspoons black pepper
2 (6-ounce) cans tomato paste
2 (14-ounce) bottles catsup
1½ teaspoons garlic salt
1 tablespoon onion salt

Brown hamburger meat and drain. Add water and boil 30 minutes. Add remaining ingredients and simmer 4-6 hours.

Bonnie B. Fleming
Clear Spring Church
Simpsonville, SC

FIESTA CHILI

- 1 pound lean ground turkey
- 1 (14½-ounce) can no-salt tomatoes
- 1 (15-ounce) can red kidney beans
- 1 (15¼-ounce) can whole kernel corn
- 1 medium onion, chopped
- 2 tablespoons chili powder
- 1 (6-ounce) can tomato paste
- 1 (6-ounce) can water
- 1 (4½-ounce) can chopped green chiles, drained
- ¾ cup Healthy Choice Fat-Free Cheddar Cheese

Brown turkey and drain. Add other ingredients except cheese and cook on medium heat for 1 hour. Serve topped with Cheddar cheese.

Lucille G. O'Donald
Burning Bush Baptist
Ringgold, GA

CHICKEN CHILI

- 3 boneless skinless chicken breasts
- 1 large onion, chopped
- 1 teaspoon seasoned salt
- 1 teaspoon garlic powder
- ½ stick butter or margarine
- 4 (15.8-ounce) cans Northern beans, undrained
- 2 (10-ounce) cans green chiles and tomatoes, undrained

In large Dutch Oven, place chicken and just enough water to cover. Add onion, seasoned salt, garlic powder, and butter. Boil chicken until it falls apart, adding water if necessary. Make sure to skim foam from top of water continually. When chicken is tender lower heat. Remove each chicken breast. Do not drain. Pull each breast apart with fingers and add back to water with heat on medium. Add beans and tomatoes with juice. Allow to simmer for at least 20 minutes. Serve with shredded cheese.

For extra spicy, use 1 can regular and 1 can of extra hot tomatoes and green chiles.

Rudy McCord
Bethel Baptist Church
Dothan, AL

'RIGINAL POTATO CHEESE SOUP

6 cups cubed potatoes
4 cups water or to cover
1 chopped onion
½ cup chopped celery or ½ teaspoon celery seed
Salt and pepper to taste
8 ounce loaf processed cheese
8 ounce carton sour cream

Cook all ingredients, except for cheese and sour cream, until potatoes are tender. Add cheese and turn stove down to simmer. When cheese is melted add sour cream and heat through. Do not boil.

Serve with cornbread or crackers

Patricia Robinson
Bowdon, GA

CHEESE SOUP

2 (10½-ounce) cans chicken broth and enough water to make 1 quart liquid
1 cup chopped onions
1 cup chopped celery
2½ cups hash browns
1 cup shredded carrot
Salt and pepper to taste
1 pound Velveeta cheese

Cook chicken broth, onion and celery for 20 minutes, then add hash browns, carrots, salt and pepper. Cook 20 minutes more and add cheese. Stir until melted.

Floria Miller
First Baptist Church
Waynesboro, GA

LOUISIANA CHICKEN GUMBO

1 chicken
1 chopped onion
2 stalks celery
1 small bell pepper, chopped
2 cloves garlic, chopped
1 bunch green onions, chopped
2 links chopped, cooked, smoked sausage
2 tablespoons Savoie's Roux
Salt and pepper to taste

Boil chicken, cool, de-bone, and chop up. Return to chicken broth along with other ingredients. Season with salt, black and red pepper to taste. Serve over rice.

Stella Sasser
Philadelphia Baptist Church
Deville, LA

MEXICAN CHICKEN SOUP

4 skinned and boned chicken breasts
1 large onion
1 tablespoon vegetable oil
2 (10-ounce) cans tomatoes and green chiles
1 (10-ounce) can Ro-tel Mexican Festival tomatoes and green chiles
1 (15½-ounce) can red kidney beans, rinsed and drained
1 (15-ounce) can black beans, rinsed and drained
1 (15¼-ounce) can whole kernel corn, drained
2 (16-ounce) cans chicken broth
1½ tablespoons chili powder
1 teaspoon sugar
½ teaspoon salt
Fresh cilantro (if desired)
Salt and pepper to taste

Cut chicken into bite sizes and chop onion into large pan. Sauté in hot oil over medium heat until chicken is lightly browned. Stir in remaining ingredients. Bring to boil over medium heat, stirring often. Cover, reduce heat and simmer 30 minutes. Sprinkle with fresh cilantro, if desired.

14 cups

Ruth Huddlest
Pleasant Grove Baptist C
Coal

BAKED POTATO SOUP

4 large potatoes
⅔ cup butter
⅔ cup flour
1½ quarts milk
Salt and pepper to taste
4 green onions
1 cup sour cream
2 cups crumbled crisp cooked bacon
5 ounces grated Cheddar cheese

Bake potatoes in 350° oven until tender. Cut potatoes in half and scoop out of skin and set aside. Melt butter in saucepan. Slowly blend in flour. Gradually add milk to the butter-flour mixture, whisking constantly. Whisk in salt and pepper and simmer over low heat, stirring constantly. When milk mixture is very hot, whisk in potatoes and onions. Whisk well, add sour cream and crumbled bacon. Heat thoroughly. Add cheese and serve with crusty French Bread.

Wanda Jones
Montevallo, AL

CORN CHOWDER

5 slices bacon
1 large onion, chopped
2 cups cubed potatoes, cooked until tender
1 (15¼-ounce) can whole kernel corn
1 (14¾-ounce) can cream style corn
1 (10¾-ounce) can cream of mushroom soup
2½ cups milk
Salt and pepper to taste

Fry bacon [illegible] crisp and set aside. Sauté onions in bacon grease and drain [illegible] other ingredients and bring to a slight boil. Serve with [illegible] on top.

Shirley Patterson
Philadelphia Baptist Church
DeVille, LA

COLD CUCUMBER SOUP

- ½ cup chopped onions
- 3 tablespoons butter
- 4 cups cucumbers, peeled, seeded and grated
- ½ teaspoon wine vinegar
- 6 cups chicken stock
- 4 teaspoons instant Cream of Wheat
- Salt and pepper to taste
- Green food coloring

Sauté onion in butter, combine with cucumbers, vinegar and stock. Cook 20 minutes. Add cream of wheat and seasonings. Cook 5 minutes and add drop of green food coloring. Whip well. Cool.

Garnish with sour cream and cucumber slice. Delicious served with deviled ham sandwiches.

8 servings

Esther L. Keane
First Baptist Church
Vernon, AL

HUNGRY MAN'S STEW

- 1 pound ground beef
- ½ cup bell pepper
- ½ cup diced onion

Sauté and drain above ingredients.

- 1 (11-ounce) can white shoepeg corn
- 1 (28-ounce) can stewed tomatoes
- 1 (16-ounce) can kidney beans
- ½ teaspoon garlic
- 1 tablespoon sugar
- 1 tablespoon chili powder
- Salt and pepper to taste

Add corn, beans and tomatoes with juices and seasonings to meat mixture. Simmer 30 minutes and enjoy.

Rose Blackwell
Laurel, MS

SANTE FE SOUP

- 2 pounds ground beef
- 1 chopped onion
- 1 (15-ounce) can black beans
- 1 (15-ounce) can pinto beans
- 1 (16-ounce) can red kidney beans
- 2 (11-ounce) cans white shoepeg corn
- 1 (14½-ounce) can diced tomatoes
- 1 (10-ounce) can tomatoes and green chiles
- 2 cups water
- 2 (1¼-ounce) packages taco seasoning
- 1 (1-ounce) package dry ranch dressing

Brown meat and onions; drain fat. Add other ingredients, including all juices and simmer for 1 hour.

Makes a large amount

Judy Field
Calvary Baptist Church
Dothan, AL

COWBOY SOUP

- 1 pound ground beef
- 1 cup chopped onion
- Salt and pepper, to taste
- 1 cup diced potatoes
- 1 cup chopped cabbage
- 1 cup sliced carrots
- 1 cup chopped celery
- ½ cup uncooked rice
- 2 (14½-ounce) cans tomatoes
- 4 cups water
- ½ teaspoon basil
- ¼ teaspoon thyme
- 2 bay leaves

Brown beef and onion and drain. Combine with everything else and bring to boil. Simmer for 1½ hours.

A perfect meal for after Sunday Church.

Rowena Hodgkins
Crievewood Baptist Church
Nashville, TN

TACO SOUP

- 1 medium onion, chopped
- 2 pounds ground beef
- 1 (16-ounce) can kidney beans, undrained
- 1 (16-ounce) can hot chili beans, undrained
- 1 (4½-ounce) can chopped green chiles
- 1 (11-ounce) can Mexican style corn
- 1 (11-ounce) can shoepeg corn
- 3 (15-ounce) cans Mexican style stewed tomatoes, undrained
- 1 (1¼-ounce) package taco seasoning
- 1 (1-ounce) package dry ranch dressing mix

Brown meat and onion and drain well. Add all other ingredients and mix well. Cook on medium heat for 30 to 45 minutes or until vegetables are done.

Large crock pot works great for working girls.

10-12 servings

Patti Dell
Sawney's Creek Baptist Church
Lugoff, SC

SISTER'S LOW CAL BEAN SOUP

- 2 cups dried pintos
- 1 onion, chopped
- 1 carrot, diced
- 2 quarts water
- 2 cups V-8 cocktail juice
- 3 bay leaves
- 1 teaspoon basil
- 1 tablespoon beef bouillon
- 1 teaspoon oregano
- 1 tablespoon picante sauce

Mix all ingredients and simmer for 3 hours or until pintos are cooked. Mash with fork.

8-10 servings

Roy Hodgkins
Crievewood Baptist Church
Nashville, TN

VEGETABLE CHOWDER

- ½ cup chopped green pepper
- ½ cup chopped onion
- ¼ cup butter
- 1 cup diced potatoes
- 1 cup diced celery
- 1 cup diced cauliflower
- 1 cup diced carrots
- 1 cup diced broccoli
- 3 cups water
- 3 chicken bouillon cubes
- 1 teaspoon salt
- ¼ teaspoon pepper
- ½ cup flour
- 2 cups milk
- 1 tablespoon parsley
- 3 cups shredded Cheddar cheese

In soup kettle, sauté green pepper and onion in butter until tender. Add all vegetables, water, bouillon cubes, salt and pepper. Bring to a boil. Reduce heat and simmer 20 minutes. Combine flour and milk until smooth. Stir into pan and bring to a boil again, stirring for 2 minutes. Just before serving add cheese and stir until melted.

Winnie Nelson
First Baptist Church
Ozark, MO

BEEF AND CABBAGE SOUP

- 1 pound ground beef, browned and drained
- 1 small onion, chopped
- ½ head small cabbage, chopped
- 1 (14½-ounce) can tomatoes
- 1 (15-ounce) can tomato sauce
- 1 (15½-ounce) can red kidney beans
- 3 cans water
- 1 teaspoon salt
- 1 teaspoon basil
- 1 teaspoon oregano

All all ingredients in large pot. Cook until tender.

Linda Doherty
Decatur, AL

CABBAGE SOUP

- 1 pound sausage
- 1 pound ground chuck
- 2 (15½-ounce) cans kidney beans
- 1 (10-ounce) can Ro-Tel tomatoes
- 1 large onion, diced
- 1 teaspoon basil
- 1 tablespoon parsley
- ½ teaspoon pepper
- 1 tablespoon sugar
- salt to taste
- 1 (46-ounce) can tomato juice
- ½ head cabbage, chopped

Cook sausage and ground chuck and drain well. Mix with remaining ingredients and simmer for at least 1 hour.

Yvonne Myers
First Baptist Church
Estill, Springs, TN

CREAM OF CAULIFLOWER SOUP

- 1 head cauliflower
- 2 tablespoons minced onion
- 2 tablespoons butter
- 1 clove garlic, optional
- ¼ cup diced celery
- 2 tablespoons flour
- 1½ cups half-and-half or cream
- ¾ teaspoon salt
- ½ cup chicken broth or more, to taste
- ¼ teaspoon nutmeg
- White pepper to taste

Trim cauliflower and break into florets. Boil 15 minutes or until tender and drain. Reserve ¾ cup florets. Puree remainder in blender. Melt butter; sauté onion, celery, and minced garlic. Stir in flour to form a smooth paste. Add milk, chicken broth, reserved cauliflower, salt, pepper and nutmeg. Heat to boiling, but do not boil.

Sarah Kerr
Holly Grove Baptist Church
Brownsville, TN

ELBOW MACARONI STEW

- 1 pound ground beef, browned and drained
- 1 onion, chopped
- 1 clove garlic, minced
- 1 (14½-ounce) can chopped tomatoes
- 1 (6-ounce) can tomato paste
- 3 cans water
- ½ bell pepper, chopped
- 1 tablespoon ground hot pepper
- Salt and pepper, to taste

Cook macaroni according to directions. Add other ingredients and simmer on low for 1 hour or until ready to serve.

Shirley Peay
St. George Baptist Church
Orangeburg, SC

TOMATO SOUP

- 1 (14½-ounce) crushed tomatoes
- ½ can water
- ½ can evaporated milk
- 3 tablespoons butter
- Salt and pepper, to taste

Bring tomatoes to slow boil and reduce heat. Add other ingredients and heat through.

Iragene Archambeault
Cobbtown, GA

OYSTER STEW (MODIFIED VERSION)

2 tablespoons margarine
½ cup chopped celery
1½ pints oysters with liquid
2 cups evaporated skim milk
¼ teaspoon salt
⅛ teaspoon black pepper
2 tablespoons parsley

In top half of a double boiler, melt margarine and sauté chopped celery for two minutes. Add oysters with liquid, evaporated skim milk, salt and pepper. Place on top of double boiler (with boiling water). Stew is done when milk is hot and oysters float and have curly edges. Garnish with parsley.

4 cups

Wanda Jones
Montevallo, AL

SHRIMP AND OKRA GUMBO

1½ pounds deveined shrimp
1 quart smothered okra
1 tablet Roux
1 cup chopped onions
1 cup chopped bell pepper
2 quarts shrimp stock
Salt and pepper, to taste

Boil shrimp shells 15 minutes to make a stock in 2 quarts water. Add roux to stock. When roux is dissolved, add cooked okra, onions and bell pepper and cook for 20 minutes. Add shrimp and continue cooking for 30 minutes. Adjust thickness with water as you like it. Pour over hot rice in bowls. Enjoy.

Gayle David
Northside Baptist Church
Lafayette, LA

EASY TURKEY STEW

- 5 pounds potatoes, cubed and chopped
- 1 large onion, chopped finely
- 8 cups canned tomatoes
- 3 (15¼-ounce) cans whole kernel corn
- 1½ pounds cooked turkey, chopped

Combine potatoes and onion in a large pot. Add water to cover top of potatoes. Cook covered until potatoes are tender. Add tomatoes and corn, bring to simmer and add the turkey. Heat to serving temperature.

Serve with hot cornbread

8-10 servings

Jeanette Statom
Westlawn Baptist Church
Huntsville, AL

CABBAGE-PINEAPPLE SLAW

- 1 (8-ounce) can unsweetened pineapple tidbits
- 3 cups finely shredded cabbage
- 1½ cups unpeeled chopped red delicious apples
- ½ cup chopped celery
- ¼ cup raisins
- ¼ cup fat-free mayonnaise

Drain pineapple; reserve juice. Combine pineapple and next 4 ingredients. Combine juice and mayonnaise. Add to cabbage and toss gently. Cover and chill.

Lucille O'Donald
Burning Bush Baptist
Ringgold, GA

CONGEALED SALAD

- 1 (6-ounce) package black raspberry or grape Jell-O
- 2 cups boiling water
- 1 (20-ounce) can crushed pineapple, drained
- 1 (16-ounce) can blueberry pie filling

Dissolve Jell-O in boiling water and add pineapple and blueberry pie filling. Place in large mold or 9 x 13 inch dish and chill in refrigerator until set. Then top with:

- 1 (8-ounce) carton sour cream
- 1 (8-ounce) package cream cheese
- ⅓ cup sugar
- 1 teaspoon vanilla

Beat well and place on top of Jell-O.

Annice McCrory
Parkway Baptist Church
Kosciusko, MS

PINK FLUFF SALAD

- 1 (20-ounce) can crushed pineapple
- 1 (16-ounce) can cherry pie filling
- 1 (14-ounce) can sweetened condensed milk
- 1 (8-ounce) carton sour cream
- 1 (10-ounce) carton frozen whipped topping
- 1 cup chopped pecans

Drain pineapple. Mix all ingredients together well. Pour into dish and chill.

This may be frozen in individual servings for serving at later time.

Lallage Seale
Pleasant Ridge Baptist Church
Hueytown, AL

ROBBY'S PINK STUFF

1 (16-ounce) carton cottage cheese
1 (3-ounce) box dry Jell-O gelatin (any flavor)
1 (14-ounce) can crushed pineapple, drained
1 small bag miniature marshmallows
1 (8-ounce) carton Cool Whip

Mix Jell-O and cottage cheese. Add other ingredients. Chill several hours or overnight.

10-12 servings

Elizabeth O'Briant
Parkway Baptist Church
Kosciusko, MS

FLUFFY FRUIT SALAD

2 (20-ounce) cans crushed pineapple
⅔ cup sugar
2 tablespoons all-purpose flour
2 eggs, slightly beaten
¼ cup orange juice
3 tablespoons lemon juice
1 tablespoon vegetable oil
2 (15¼-ounce) cans fruit cocktail, drained
2 (11-ounce) cans mandarin oranges, drained
2 bananas, sliced
1 cup heavy cream, whipped

Drain pineapple, reserving 1 cup juice and set pineapple aside. In small sauce pan add juice, sugar, flour, eggs, orange juice, and oil; bring to a boil, stirring constantly. Boil for 1 minute, remove from heat and let cool. In a salad bowl combine pineapple, fruit cocktail, oranges and bananas. Fold in the whipped cream and cooled sauce. Chill several hours before serving.

Marguerite Dinkins
Sawney's Creek Baptist Church
Ridgeway, SC

LOW SODIUM CHICKEN SALAD

1 cooked chicken
1 cup celery
1 teaspoon black pepper
2 dashes cayenne
½ cup light mayonnaise
¼ cup vinegar
¼ teaspoon garlic powder
2 boiled eggs
Pickles, if desired
Salt and pepper, to taste

Chop chicken, celery and eggs. Add all ingredients together and refrigerate.

Helen Rhyne
Calvary Baptist Church
Lincolnton, NC

COLORFUL CHICKEN SALAD

2 cups chicken breasts, cooked and cubed
¼ cup finely diced celery
¼ cup golden raisins
¼ cup dried cranberries
¼ cup sliced almonds
¾ cup mayonnaise
2 tablespoons chopped red onion
¼ teaspoon salt
¼ teaspoon pepper

In bowl combine all ingredients. Mix well and refrigerate.

2 cups or 4 sandwiches

This recipe is great for serving at showers, bridal teas, etc. Just spoon about 1 heaping teaspoon into small tarts. They are wonderful.

Jeanette Statom
Westlawn Baptist Church
Huntsville, AL

CHICKEN SALAD

- 6 chicken breasts
- 3 eggs, boiled and chopped
- 3 celery stalks, chopped
- 1 teaspoon salt
- ½ teaspoon pepper
- 1 medium onion, chopped
- 1 cup chopped grapes
- 1 cup chopped pecans
- ½ cup mayonnaise

Cook chicken until tender. Chop into small pieces, Add other ingredients, adding mayonnaise last.

To make moister, you may want to add more mayonnaise.

Shirley Morgan
Faith Baptist Church
Trinity, AL

HOT CHICKEN SALAD

- 8 boneless chicken breasts
- 1 cup chopped celery
- ½ cup chopped onion
- 1 (10¾-ounce) can cream of mushroom soup
- 1 cup Hellmann's mayonnaise
- 1 (8-ounce) can sliced water chestnuts, drained
- 1 package Pepperidge Farm dressing mix
- 1 stick margarine

After cooking and cutting up chicken, add all ingredients except for dressing mix and margarine. Mix well and put in 9 x 13 inch baking dish. Melt margarine and add to dressing mix and spread over top of chicken mixture. Bake in 350° oven for 35 to 40 minutes or until hot and bubbly.

Elsie Lobb
Greenfield, IN

CURRIED CHICKEN SALAD

- 4 cups diced, cooked chicken breasts
- ¾ cup mayonnaise
- 1 teaspoon curry powder
- ½ cup finely chopped celery
- ¼ cup finely chopped onion
- 1 (8-ounce) can crushed pineapple, drained
- 1 large apple, finely chopped
- ½ cup golden raisins

Mix mayonnaise and curry powder together. Mix all ingredients together and keep refrigerated.

Carolyn Hartley
First Baptist Church
Palmerdale, AL

ORANGE TAPIOCA SALAD

- 3 cups water
- 1 (3-ounce) package orange Jell-O
- 1 (3.4-ounce) package instant vanilla pudding mix
- 1 (3.4-ounce) package tapioca pudding mix
- 1 (11-ounce) can mandarin oranges
- 1 (8-ounce) can crushed pineapple, drained
- 1 (10-ounce) carton frozen whipped topping

In sauce pan, bring water to boil. Whisk in Jell-O and pudding mixes. Return to boil, stirring constantly; boil for 1 minute. Remove from heat and cool completely. Fold in oranges, pineapple and whipped topping. Spoon into serving bowl, cover and chill for at least 2 hours.

12-14 servings

Ginevieve Hagy
Harlan, KY

ORANGE SALAD

- 2 (3.4-ounce) packages orange Jell-O
- 2 cups boiling water
- 1 (6-ounce) can frozen orange juice
- 2 (11-ounce) cans mandarin oranges, drained
- 1 (20-ounce) can crushed pineapple, with juice
- 1 (10-ounce) carton frozen whipped topping
- 1 (3.4-ounce) package lemon instant pudding mix
- 1 cup milk

Dissolve Jell-O in boiling water. Add frozen juice and stir until melted. Add oranges and pineapple. Pour into 9 x 13 inch dish and chill until set. Mix milk with pudding mix and fold in whipped topping. Spread on top of congealed mixture and refrigerate.

Marion Bannister
Clear Spring Baptist Church.

RED HOT JELL-O SALAD

- 1 (3-ounce) box cherry Jell-O
- 1 (12-ounce) can 7-Up
- ¼ cup red hots
- 1 cup applesauce

Heat 7-Up to boiling in medium pan. Stir and dissolve red hots in 7-Up. Pour hot mixture over Jell-O granules in bowl and stir until dissolved. Add applesauce and stir until smooth. Chill until set.

Jeanne Jeffries

JELL-O SALAD

- 1 (3-ounce) package apricot Jell-O
- 1 cup water
- 1 (11-ounce) can mandarin oranges
- 1 cup small marshmallows
- 1 cup sour cream
- ½ cup chopped pecans
- 1 cup coconut

Boil water and juice from oranges and mix with Jell-O. Mix other ingredients until well mixed. Pour into mold and refrigerate. Serve with lettuce and Cool Whip.

Virginia Hern
Porter Memorial Baptist Church
Lexington, KY

ANNIE MAE FROST'S FRUIT SALAD

- 1 lemon, squeezed
- 1 (20-ounce) can sliced pineapple
- ¾ cup sugar
- 1 tablespoon flour
- 3 eggs
- 1 yellow apple
- 3 bananas
- ½ cup chopped pecans

Mix sugar and flour in boiled. Add lemon juice and ¾ of the juice from pineapple can. Beat eggs and add to above mixture. Cook on medium heat until thick. Cool sauce well and add 7 slices pineapple (cut up), sliced bananas, chopped apple and pecans. Chill and serve.

Ethel Freeman
West Monroe, LA

FRUITY FRUIT SALAD

1 (20-ounce) can chunk pineapple
1 (15¼-ounce) can mixed fruit (chunky)
2 bananas
3 tablespoons Tang
1 (5.1-ounce) box vanilla instant pudding mix

Drain fruit well. Save juice from pineapple. Mix pineapple juice with vanilla pudding and tang. Pour over fruit and chill.

Jean Leonard
Indian Lake Baptist Church
Northport, AL

FROZEN FRUIT SALAD

1 (8-ounce) package cream cheese
1 (14-ounce) can sweetened condensed milk
1 (8-ounce) can crushed pineapple
1 (16-ounce) can cherry pie mix
1 (10-ounce) carton frozen whipped topping

Soften cream cheese and mix with milk. Add other ingredients and put in dish and freeze until 1 hour before eating.

Leoneve Whitmire
Lakewood Baptist
Gainesville, GA

BLUEBERRY SALAD

- 2 (3-ounce) packages black raspberry Jell-O
- 2 cups boiling water
- 1 (15-ounce) can blueberries
- 1 (8-ounce) can crushed pineapple
- 1 (8-ounce) package cream cheese
- ½ cup sugar
- ½ pint sour cream
- ½ cup chopped pecans
- ½ teaspoon vanilla

Dissolve Jell-O in boiling water. Drain blueberries and pineapple and measure liquid. Add water to make 1 cup and add to Jell-O mixture. Stir in blueberries and pineapple. Pour into 2-quart container. Cover and refrigerate until firm. Combine cream cheese, sugar, sour cream and vanilla and spread over congealed salad. May sprinkle with pecans, if desired.

10-12 servings

Neola Cleveland
First Baptist Church
Booneville, MC

FRUIT SALAD

- 1 (16-ounce) can peach pie filling
- 1 (15¼-ounce) can pineapple tidbits, drained
- 1 banana, sliced
- 1 cup green grapes, sliced
- 1 (16-ounce) jar maraschino cherries, drained
- 2 kiwi, peeled and sliced
- 1 (10-ounce) carton Cool Whip

Mix all ingredients together. Cover with Cool Whip and chill.

Gertie Key
Fellowship Baptist
Mt. Airy, NC

BEAN SALAD

- 1 (14½-ounce) can French style green beans
- 1 (15-ounce) can green peas
- 1 (11-ounce) can white shoepeg corn
- 1 (2-ounce) jar chopped pimento
- ½ cup chopped onion
- ½ cup chopped bell pepper
- 1 cup sugar
- ½ teaspoon pepper
- 1 teaspoon salt
- ½ cup oil
- ¾ cup vinegar

Combine vegetables and set aside. Combine rest of ingredients in a saucepan and heat. Stir often until all ingredients are dissolved. Pour over vegetables. Stir gently, cover and chill for 24 hours.

Cassie Mayfield
Simpsonville, SC

CAULIFLOWER SALAD

- 1 cup mayonnaise
- ¼ cup sugar
- 1 large head iceberg lettuce
- 7 slices crisp bacon
- ½ head cauliflower
- ¼ cup Parmesan cheese

Mix mayonnaise and sugar together at least 3 hours before serving and refrigerate. Tear lettuce into bite-size pieces and crumble bacon into lettuce. Cut or break cauliflower into small pieces and add. Toss and mix with dressing just before serving. Top with Parmesan.

Nancy Walker
Precision Valley Baptist
Springfield, VT

BROCCOLI AND CAULIFLOWER SALAD

1 head cauliflower
1 bunch broccoli
½ green pepper
1 small red onion
1 cup Kraft Miracle Whip
½ cup sugar
⅓ cup vinegar
⅓ cup oil

Cut vegetables into small pieces. Thoroughly mix Miracle Whip, sugar, vinegar and oil and toss with vegetables. Chill and serve

Jocie Flint
First Baptist Church
Henderson, KY

CHERRY SALAD

1 (16-ounce) can cherry pie filling
1 (20-ounce) can crushed pineapple, drained
1 cup chopped nuts
1 cup miniature marshmallows
1 (14-ounce) can condensed milk
1 (12-ounce) carton Cool Whip

Mix lightly with a fork. Do not stir. You may reserve some of the cherries from the pie filling to put on top if desired.

Dean Smith
Derma Baptist Church
Calhoun City, MS

FIVE CUP SALAD

1 cup mandarin oranges
1 cup pineapple, crushed
1 cup miniature marshmallows
1 cup coconut
1 cup cottage cheese

Drain oranges and pineapple. Mix all ingredients and refrigerate overnight.

Ruby Shumpert
West Cola, SC

PEAR SALAD

1 (16-ounce) can pears (light syrup)
1 (3-ounce) package lemon Jell-O (no sugar)
1 (8-ounce) package low fat cream cheese
1 cup chopped pecans (optional)
1 cup low-fat Cool Whip

Drain pears, reserving liquid. Add water to liquid to make 1 cup. Bring liquid to boil, remove from heat and add Jell-O. Chill until partially set. While this is chilling, blend pears and cream cheese until creamy. When Jell-O is beginning to thicken, stir in the pear-cheese mixture. Add pecans and fold in Cool Whip. Place in mold and refrigerate until set.

Loreva Sparks
New Chapel Hill Baptist
Calhoun, LA

CORNBREAD SALAD

1 (8½-ounce) package jalapeño cornbread mix
2 fresh tomatoes, diced
2 small green peppers, diced
1 small onion, diced
¾ cup mayonnaise
1 cup grated cheese
1 cup ham diced

Bake cornbread as per directions on package. Cool, crumble and add all the above ingredients. Chill before using.

If you don't have ham you can use bacon, turkey or sausage.

Carolyn Mace
Amboy Baptist Church
North Little Rock, AR

POTATO SALAD

3 cups cubed, cooked and cooled potatoes
1 tablespoon minced onion
1 teaspoon salt
¼ cup chopped green peppers
¼ cup finely cut celery
1 medium tomato, cubed
2 hard-boiled eggs, chopped
½ cup salad dressing
Paprika, to taste

Combine all ingredients and toss lightly. Sprinkle with paprika and chill.

Ruby Isenberg
Crosspointe Baptist Church
Owensboro, KY

APPLE SALAD

⅓ cup plain flour
¾ cup sugar
1 (12-ounce) carton whipping cream
1 (20-ounce) can crushed pineapple, undrained
½ stick margarine
1 cup chopped pecans
4 large apples, chopped

Mix flour and sugar well. Stir in whipping cream (unwhipped). Add pineapple and juice and heat on medium heat, stirring constantly. Remove from heat and add margarine. Let cool and add chopped apples and nuts to cooked mixture and mix well. Serve warm or cold.

Bessie H. Whaley
Fairview Heights Northside Church
Anniston, AL

YUM YUM SALAD

1 (16-ounce) can fruit cocktail
1 (11-ounce) can mandarin oranges
1 (8-ounce) can pineapple
1 (3.4-ounce) package lemon Jell-O
½ cup coconut
1 cup miniature marshmallows
½ cup nuts
Any fruits you desire (optional)

Combine all ingredients (along with juices) and refrigerate.

Jane Howard
Sweeny, TX

HAM AND MACARONI SALAD

- ½ pound boiled or baked ham
- ½ cup diced Cheddar cheese
- 2 cups cooked elbow macaroni
- 1 cup chopped celery
- 2 small onions, chopped
- ½ cup diced dill pickle
- ½ cup mayonnaise
- 2 teaspoons prepared mustard

Dice ham into ½-inch cubes. Combine ham and cheese with macaroni, celery, onion and pickle. Mix mayonnaise and mustard, then stir into macaroni mixture and mix well. Chill until ready to serve.

4 servings

Norma Burgess
Skyline Heights Baptist Church
Johnson City, TN

CRANBERRY SALAD

- 1 (14-ounce) can whole cranberry sauce
- 1 (8-ounce) can crushed pineapple
- 1 (3-ounce) package strawberry or cherry Jell-O
- 1 cup nuts

Mix all ingredients. Refrigerate and serve.

Mary Lee King
First Baptist Church
Avon Park, FL

GRAPE SALAD

2 pounds red seedless grapes
2 pounds green seedless grapes
1 (8-ounce) package cream cheese
1 (8-ounce) package sour cream
½ cup sugar
1 teaspoon vanilla
1 cup brown sugar
1 cup chopped pecans

Cream sour cream, cream cheese, sugar and vanilla in a large serving bowl. Fold grapes into mixture. Top with brown sugar and chopped pecans. Refrigerate.

Hazel Perry
Lineville Baptist Church
Lineville, AL

JACK LEVERETT'S CONGEALED SALAD FOR DIABETICS

1 (5-ounce) package sugar-free raspberry Jell-O
1 (8-ounce) can unsweetened crushed pineapple, drained
1 (14-ounce) can whole cranberry sauce
1 cup chopped pecans
1½ cups boiling water

Put cranberry sauce and pineapple in refrigerator ahead of preparation time to chill well. To prepare: mix Jell-O with boiling water. Add drained pineapple and cranberry sauce and pecans. Stir until well mixed. Refrigerate until firm.

Rachel H. Ayer
Christ United Methodist
Forsyth, GA

MACARONI SALAD

- ½ cup chopped onion
- ½ cup bell pepper, chopped
- 2 tablespoons oil
- 1 pound Velveeta cheese
- ½ cup milk
- 2 cups cooked macaroni
- ½ cup Parmesan cheese

Sauté onion and bell pepper in oil, add cheese and melt, then add milk. Add cooked macaroni and pour into 9 x 13 inch casserole dish. Top with Parmesan cheese and cook 20 minutes at 350°.

Yvonne Sherrill
Spruce Pine, AL

SPAGHETTI SALAD

- 1 (16-ounce) package thin spaghetti
- 1 (16-ounce) bottle Italian dressing
- ½ bottle Salad Supreme seasoning
- 2 large tomatoes, diced
- 1 large red onion, diced
- 1 large green pepper, chopped
- 2 avocados (if desired) chopped

Cook spaghetti and drain. Add chopped onions and peppers and Salad Supreme. Pour Italian dressing over mixture, stir and marinate over night. Add tomatoes just before serving. Makes a large bowl.

Bobbie Webber
First Baptist Church
Lake Jackson, TX

STRAWBERRY PRETZEL SALAD

- 2 cups pretzels, broken
- 1 tablespoon sugar
- 1½ sticks butter, melted
- 1 (8-ounce) package cream cheese
- 1 cup sugar
- 1 (10-ounce) carton frozen whipped topping
- 2 (10-ounce) packages frozen strawberries, thawed
- 2 cups boiling water
- 1 (5-ounce) package strawberry Jell-O

Mix pretzels, 1 tablespoon sugar and butter together and spread in 9 x 13 inch dish. Bake at 450° for 8 minutes. Let cool. Cream sugar and cream cheese and fold in whipped topping. Layer on top of cooled crust. Mix Jell-O, water and strawberries. Refrigerate to let cool (do not let congeal) then pour over top of mixture, chill and serve.

Myrtle Campbell
Calvary Baptist Church
Dothan, AL

PEA SALAD

- 1 (8½-ounce) can LeSueur peas
- 1 cup shredded sharp Cheddar cheese
- 1 cup chopped celery
- ½ cup chopped green onions
- 4 sweet pickles, chopped
- ½ cup chopped pecans
- 2 tablespoons salad dressing
- Salt and pepper, to taste

Mix all ingredients and chill.

Nice crunchy, crisp salad, keeps well.

Jewell Overton
Holly Grove Baptist Church
Bells, TN

GOLDEN GLOW SALAD

- 2 (3-ounce) packages orange Jell-O
- 2 cups boiling water
- ¾ cup sugar
- 1 cup grated carrots
- ½ cup grated cheese
- 1 (20-ounce) can crushed pineapple and juice
- 1 (12-ounce) carton frozen whipped topping

Mix Jell-O, water and sugar and stir until dissolved. Chill until thick. Add carrots, cheese and pineapple with juice and stir well; chill more, (do not let set hard). Fold in whipped topping. Return to refrigerator until ready to serve.

Susie Hayes
Holly Grove Baptist Church
Bells, TN

CABBAGE SALAD

- 1 cabbage head, chopped
- ½ green pepper, diced
- 1-2 carrots, grated
- Salt, to taste
- 1 cup sugar
- ½ cup oil
- 1 cup white vinegar
- ½ cup water

Mix cabbage, pepper, carrots and salt. Mix sugar, oil, vinegar and water and pour over cabbage mixture. This can be used immediately or better to let chill overnight. Will keep indefinitely.

Edna Brooks
Holly Grove Baptist Church
Bells, TN

SUNSHINE SALAD

- 1 (3-ounce) package orange Jell-O
- 1 cup hot water
- 1 tablespoon vinegar
- 1 cup raw carrots, grated
- 1 teaspoon plain gelatin
- 1 (15-ounce) can crushed pineapple
- ¼ teaspoon salt

Mix plain gelatin with orange Jell-O and dissolve in hot water. Add pineapple with juice and vinegar. Season carrots with salt and add to gelatin. Turn into mold or bowl and chill until firm. Serve plain or on lettuce with mayonnaise.

6-8 servings

Frances Tate
Parkwood Baptist Church
Concord, NC

CORNBREAD SALAD

- 1 medium pan cornbread
- 1 medium green pepper, chopped
- 1 medium onion, chopped
- 1 medium tomato, cut into small pieces
- ½ cup cubed sharp Cheddar cheese
- 1 tablespoon sugar
- 1 tablespoon mustard
- ½ cup mayonnaise

Cook and crumble cornbread. Mix other ingredients and add to cornbread.

Serve with pinto beans or potato soup.

Annette Zirbel
Wooley Springs Baptist Church
Athens, AL

CRAB SALAD

- 1 (6½-ounce) can white crabmeat
- ½ cup grated sharp Cheddar cheese
- 1 egg, hard-boiled and chopped
- ¼ cup finely chopped celery
- 2 tablespoons chopped green onion
- 2 tablespoons sweet pickle relish
- 3 tablespoons mayonnaise
- ¼ teaspoon lemon juice
- ½ teaspoon horse radish
- Salt and pepper, to taste

Mix all ingredients and chill.

Catherine Carter
Westwood Baptist Church
Alabaster, AL

SUMMER SALAD

- 1 chicken, cooked and chopped
- 1 apple, chopped
- 1 cup grapes, chopped
- ½ cup pecans, chopped
- ½ cup sour cream
- ½ cup mayonnaise

Blend all ingredients together and chill.

Serve with Ritz Crackers

Sylvia Hill
Danville, AL

KRAUT SALAD

- 1 cup chopped onions
- 1 cup chopped sweet pepper
- ⅓ cup chopped celery
- 1 cup sugar
- ¾ cup vinegar
- 1 (14½-ounce) can chopped kraut

Mix onions, peppers, celery, sugar and vinegar together, blending well, add kraut and chill.

Carolyn Maddox
Holly Grove Baptist Church
Brownsville, TN

SHRIMP MACARONI SALAD

1 cup quick cooking macaroni
1 cup chopped celery
1 small onion, chopped
¼ cup chopped pimento
¼ cup French dressing
1½ cups cooked shrimp
2 hard-boiled eggs, chopped
½ teaspoon salt
¼ teaspoon paprika
¼ cup chopped green pepper
1 cup mayonnaise

Cook macaroni in boiling, salted water about 7 minutes or until tender. Chill and add celery, onion, green pepper, pimento, shrimp, eggs and seasonings and mix. Moisten with mayonnaise and French dressing. Serve on lettuce. Garnish with hard-boiled eggs.

6 servings

Rupel McInnish
Bethel Baptist Church
Dothan, AL

AFTER THE HOLIDAYS SALAD

2 cups turkey, diced
1 cup pineapple chunks, well drained
1 cup diced celery
½ cup sliced green onion
¼ cup dry roasted peanuts
1 cup seedless green grapes
⅔ cup mayonnaise
2 tablespoons chopped chutney
1 tablespoon lime juice
½ teaspoon curry powder
¼ teaspoon salt
Lettuce leaves, optional

In a mixing bowl, toss turkey, pineapple, celery, green onions, peanuts and grapes. In small bowl, combine remaining ingredients except lettuce. Pour over turkey mixture and mix gently. Chill. Serve on bed of lettuce.

4 servings

Gail Doe
Westwood Baptist Church
Alabaster, AL

DERBY SALAD

- 1 (12-ounce) can condensed milk
- ¼ cup lemon juice
- 1 (10-ounce) carton Cool Whip
- 3 bananas, sliced
- 1 cup miniature marshmallows
- 1 (20-ounce) can crushed pineapple, drained

Mix condensed milk and lemon juice together well. Stir in other ingredients and refrigerate.

Jean Claunch
Salvisa, KY

APPLE-SNICKERS BAR SALAD

- 6 Granny Smith apples
- 1 (10-ounce) carton frozen whipped topping
- 6 Snickers candy bars
- 1 (8-ounce) carton sour cream

Dice apples. Cut candy bars into small pieces. Mix apples, candy, whipped topping and sour cream. Let set overnight in refrigerator.

Louise Grimme
Ozark, MO

JURASSIC PARK COLE SLAW

- 1 head cabbage
- 8 ounces mixed crystallized fruit
- ½ cup dried cranberries
- 1 cup sugar
- 1 teaspoon salt
- 2 tablespoons chopped onion
- 1 ounce salad oil
- 1 tablespoon paprika
- 1 tablespoon Dijon mustard
- 8 ounces apple cider vinegar

Shred cabbage and add fruit and cranberries; toss together and set aside. Whisk remaining ingredients together until blended well. Pour over cabbage mixture when ready to serve.

Prepare cabbage mixture and dressing the night before serving and store in separate bags in the refrigerator. The day of serving pour dressing over cabbage mixture and mix well. Great with Bar-B-Que.

Jeanette Statom
Westlawn Baptist Church
Huntsville, AL

PIZZA SALAD

- 2 cans Pillsbury crescent rolls
- 1 (1-ounce) package dry ranch dressing mix
- 1 cup mayonnaise
- 2 (8-ounce) packages cream cheese
- Desired amounts of fresh vegetables cut into small pieces

Roll out crescent rolls onto baking sheet making one piece. Bake for 8 minutes at temperature on package. Mix all other ingredients except vegetables and spread over cooled crescent rolls; top with vegetables and cut into small pieces before serving.

Ruby Branham
Sawney's Creek Baptist Church
Elgin, SC

Vegetables

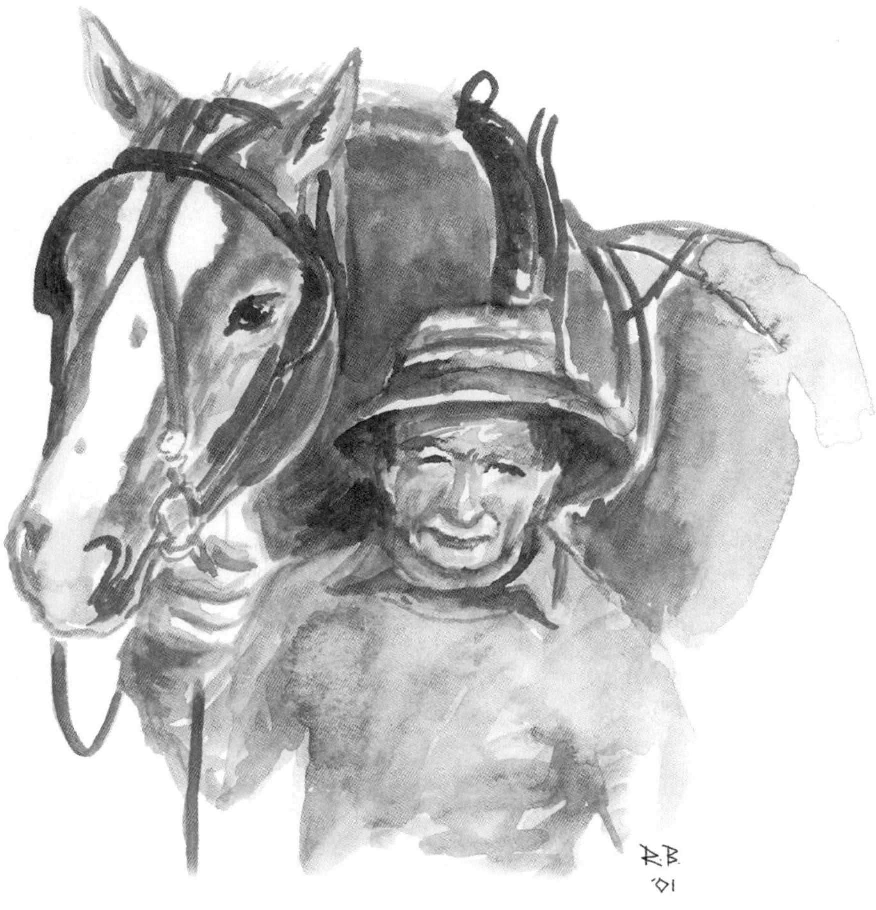

Better is a dish of vegetables where love is,
than a fattened ox and hatred with it. Proverbs 15:17

SWEET POTATO SURPRISE

- 3 cups sweet potatoes, cooked, mashed and cooled
- 1 cup sugar
- 2 eggs
- 1 tablespoon vanilla
- 1 stick melted butter
- 1 packed cup brown sugar
- ⅓ cup flour
- ⅓ cup butter, softened
- 1 cup nuts

Mix potatoes and next 3 ingredients with mixer at high speed. Place in 9 x 13 inch casserole bowl. Mix remaining ingredients together and sprinkle on top of sweet potato mixture. Bake at 350° for 30 minutes.

Mildred Williams
Second Baptist Church
Warner Robins, GA

SUNDAY SWEET POTATOES

- 3 cups sweet potatoes, mashed
- 1 cup sugar
- ½ cup milk
- ⅓ cup butter or margarine
- 2 eggs, well beaten
- 1 teaspoon vanilla
- 1 cup coconut
- 1 cup chopped nuts
- 1 cup brown sugar
- ⅓ cup flour
- ⅓ cup melted butter or margarine

Combine potatoes and next 5 ingredients and pour into 9 x 13 inch baking dish. Blend coconut, nuts, brown sugar and flour. Add butter and sprinkle over potatoes. Bake at 325° for about 20 minutes.

Ethel Styles
Locust Hill Baptist Church
Travelers Rest, SC

TRAIN WRECK SWEET POTATOES

- 1 (40-ounce) can sweet potatoes
- 1 (10-ounce) can crushed pineapple
- ½ cup brown sugar
- 2 tablespoons butter or margarine
- 1 teaspoon ground cinnamon
- Dash ground nutmeg

Heat oven to 325°. Reserve ⅓ cup liquid from potatoes. In 2-quart casserole dish that has been buttered or sprayed with nonstick cooking spray, combine sweet potatoes with ⅓ cup of liquid from potatoes, pineapple with juice, brown sugar, butter or margarine (cut into small pieces), cinnamon and nutmeg. Bake for 60 to 80 minutes, stirring occasionally, until juices become syrupy (cooks well with roasting turkey or baking ham—just stir whenever meat is basted, glazed or checked).

8 servings

Alice Lawrence
Stetson Baptist Church
Deland, FL

CANDIED SWEET POTATOES

- 2-3 medium sweet potatoes
- 1½ cups brown sugar
- 1 tablespoon flour
- ½ teaspoon salt
- ½ stick butter
- 5-6 tablespoons hot water

Boil potatoes until tender. Peel and cut lengthwise and place in a buttered baking dish. Mix brown sugar, flour and salt together in a saucepan, add butter and water, let come to a boil, and pour over potatoes. Put in oven and bake 350° for 20 to 30 minutes.

Nancy Woody
First Baptist Church,
Queen City,TX

VEGETABLE PIZZA

- 2 (8-ounce) cans crescent rolls
- 2 (8-ounce) cans nonfat cream cheese
- ¾ cup light mayonnaise
- 1 (1-ounce) package dry ranch dressing mix
- ¾ cup tomato, diced
- ¾ cup broccoli, diced
- ¾ cup cauliflower, diced
- ¾ cup green pepper, diced
- ¾ cup onion, diced
- ¾ cup mushroom, diced
- ¾ cup carrots, diced
- (You can use any kind of vegetables you like.)
- 6 ounces Cheddar cheese, grated
- 6 ounces mozzarella cheese, grated

Spray cookie sheet with cooking spray. Spread rolls on cookie sheet; pinch seams together. Bake 10 minutes at 350°. Cool completely. Mix cream cheese, mayonnaise, and ranch dressing mix together. Spread over crust. Decorate with vegetables; put tomatoes on top. Sprinkle with the cheeses and enjoy.

JoAnn Oakley
Lake Catomia Baptist
Cullman, AL

GERMAN FRIED VEGETABLES

- 1 cup diced green tomatoes
- 1 cup diced potatoes
- 1 cup diced squash
- 1 cup thinly sliced okra
- ½ cup chopped onion
- ½ cup diced bell peppers
- Salt and pepper, to taste
- Dash garlic powder
- ½ cup flour
- ½ cup meal
- 2 tablespoons vegetable oil
- 2 tablespoons butter

Toss all vegetables together. Batter with same amount of flour and meal. Fry in half shortening and half butter.

d with corn on the cob, meat loaf and cole slaw.

Betty Ross
Hanceville, AL

SPINACH BARS

1 cup flour
1 cup milk
Tabasco sauce, to taste
1 pound shredded Cheddar cheese
¼ cup melted butter
2 eggs, beaten
1 (10-ounce) package frozen spinach

Cook spinach per directions on back of package and mix with other ingredients. Pour into a greased 13 x 9 inch pan. Bake at 350° for about 30 minutes; cut in squares. May be served warm or can be frozen for later use.

Verlon Honeycutt
Joy Makers, First Baptist Church
Booneville, MS

CORN PUDDING

1½ cups fresh corn (4 to 5 ears)
4 eggs, slightly beaten
2 cups milk
½ cup saltine cracker crumbs
2 teaspoons sugar
2 teaspoons salt
⅛ teaspoon pepper
¼ cup melted butter

Cut corn from cob and scrape cob. Beat eggs. Add milk, sugar, salt, pepper, butter and corn. Stir together. Add cracker crumbs. Pour into 2½-quart casserole and place dish in a pan of water. Bake at 350° for 1 hour or until center is set.

8 servings

Marjorie Cameron
Wayside Baptist Church
Miami, FL

MICROWAVE CAULIFLOWER

Place cauliflower (whole) in microwave until nearly done (be sure it's in a covered bowl with a lid and a little water to steam). Pour off water and pour a mixture of mustard and mayonnaise (more mayonnaise than mustard) over it. Sprinkle with Cheddar cheese and paprika. Return to microwave until cheese is melted.

Rusty Hayes

FRUIT-FILLED SQUASH

- **2 small or medium acorn squash**
- **1 cup chopped apple**
- **½ cup orange, peeled and diced**
- **½ cup brown sugar**
- **½ teaspoon grated orange peel**
- **4 teaspoons butter or margarine**
- **¼ cup water**

Cut squash in half crosswise, remove seeds; sprinkle cavities with salt. Combine apple, orange, brown sugar, orange peel, and ½ teaspoon salt. Spoon into squash cavities; dot each with 1 teaspoon of the butter. Wrap each half securely in foil. Stack cut side up in crockpot. Add water; cover and cook on low heat for 6 hours. Unwrap squash and lift to serving platter. Drain any syrup remaining in foil into a small pitcher. Serve with squash.

4 servings

Edith Dockery
Providence Baptist Church
Shreveport, LA

SQUASH DRESSING

- 2 cups cooked, drained and mashed yellow squash
- 2 cups cornbread crumbs
- 1 (10¾-ounce) can cream of chicken soup
- 1 medium onion, chopped
- 1 stick margarine, melted
- 3 eggs, beaten
- Salt and pepper, to taste

Mix all ingredients together and bake at 350° for 40 to 45 minutes until firm.

Emma G. York
Prattmont Baptist Church
Prattville, AL

SPAGHETTI SQUASH SURPRISE PIE

- 4 cups of cooked, shredded spaghetti squash
- ½ cup sugar
- 8 individual packets of artificial sweetener
- Egg substitute equal to 4 eggs
- ¼ cup low calorie margarine
- ½ cup flour
- 2 cups 1% milk
- ¼ teaspoon salt
- ½ teaspoon baking powder
- 1 teaspoon vanilla
- 1 teaspoon coconut flavoring

Prepare squash by slicing lengthwise and scooping out seeds with a spoon. Place squash halves cut side down on a baking tray or cookie sheet (spray pan with cooking spray or line with foil to make clean up easier). Bake squash for 45 minutes in a 350° oven. When squash is cool to the touch, scrape inside of squash with a fork. Squash will come out in strands that look like spaghetti. Spray two 8-inch pie pans with non-stick spray and then coat with flour. Place 2 cups of squash in each pie plate. Put all remaining ingredients into a blender. Blend well. Pour equally over the squash in the two pie pans. Bake at 350° for 60 minutes. A crust will form on the bottom, pie filling is the center and the spaghetti squash (mock coconut) is the topping.

Alice Lawrence
Stetson Baptist Church
Deland, FL

BAKED SQUASH RITZ

2 pounds of yellow squash
1 onion
2 beaten eggs
1 cup evaporated milk
1 cup grated cheese
2 tablespoon butter
Salt and pepper
2 cups crushed Ritz crackers

Cook squash and onion; drain. Add remaining ingredients except crackers. Place in a greased casserole and top with crushed Ritz crackers. Bake 45 minutes to 1 hour in a 350° oven.

8 servings

Mildred Horne
Miami, FL

BATTLETOWN INN SQUASH

7 small yellow squash
1 small onion, diced
½ cup cream
¼ cup crushed saltines
1 tablespoon butter
1 cup bread crumbs

Boil squash in salted water until done. Drain and mash. Sauté onion in butter. Add cream and crackers. Combine with mashed squash. Pour into greased dish and top with bread crumbs. Dot with butter. Bake at 400° for 30 minutes.

Norma Burgess
Skyline Heights Baptist Church
Johnson City, TN

BAKED BEANS

- 1 (23-ounce) can pork and beans
- 1 large onion, chopped
- ¼ large green pepper, chopped
- 2 tablespoons vegetable cooking oil
- ½ cup molasses
- ½ cup brown sugar
- 2 tablespoons mustard
- Black pepper, to taste

Over medium heat, cook onion and green pepper until onion is transparent. Place beans in large casserole dish. Add brown sugar, molasses and mustard. Mix; add onion-pepper mixture and black pepper. Mix well. Cook at 350° for 1 hour.

Merle Cable
Pleasant Garden Baptist Church
Pleasant Garden, NC

PARTY POTATOES

- 1 (27-ounce) package hash brown potatoes
- 1 cup cream of mushroom soup
- 1 cup cream of chicken soup
- 2 cups processed cheese product, cubed
- ½ cup onion, chopped
- ½ cup sour cream

Combine all ingredients. Pour into 9 x 13 inch pan. Bake at 350° for 20 to 35 minutes.

Dorothy Kelly
First Baptist Church
Ozark, MO

PARTY POTATOES

- 12 medium potatoes
- ½ pound processed cheese product, cubed
- 4 slices bread, cubed
- 1 small onion, diced
- 2 sticks butter, cut up
- 1 cup milk
- 1 teaspoon parsley
- ¼ teaspoon pepper
- Cornflake crumbs

Boil potatoes with skins on. Take skins off potatoes and cube. Mix everything together. Pour into a 9 x 13 inch baking dish. Sprinkle top with cornflake crumbs. Bake at 350° for 45 minutes.

If you want to cut the recipe in half it does not take as long to cook.

Catherine Carter
Westwood Baptist
Alabaster, AL

DELICIOUS SCALLOPED POTATOES

- 6 cups sliced potatoes
- Salt and pepper, to taste
- 1 onion
- 2 tablespoons butter
- 1¼ cups processed cheese product or Cheddar cheese soup
- 1 (10¾-ounce) can cream of mushroom soup
- ½ cup milk

Cook potatoes until almost done. Salt and pepper to taste. Cook onion with 2 tablespoons butter. Layer potatoes, onions, and cheese in a 9 x 13 inch baking dish. Top with soup and bake until bubbly and brown.

You may also use water chestnuts, pimento, ham or bacon.

Judy Morisset
First Baptist Church
Ozark, MO

PARTY POTATOES

8-10 medium potatoes
1 (8-ounce) package cream cheese
1 (8-ounce) carton sour cream
4 tablespoons butter or margarine
⅓ cup chopped chives
Salt and pepper, to taste
Paprika

Boil potatoes until tender. Beat sour cream and cream cheese together. Add hot potatoes and beat until smooth. Add butter, chives, salt and pepper. Pour into well greased 2-quart casserole dish. Dot with butter and sprinkle paprika on top. Bake at 350° for 25 minutes.

8-10 servings

Laura Bolick
Lincolnton, NC

HASH BROWN AU GRATIN

2 pounds frozen hash brown potatoes
½ cup melted butter
Salt and pepper
¼ cup chopped onions
1 (10¾-ounce) can cream of chicken soup
1 (8-ounce) carton sour cream
2 cups grated Cheddar cheese

Mix well-place in a 9 x 13 inch baking dish. Top with bread crumbs. Bake at 350° for 45 minutes.

Grace Tarrant
The Chapel at Lake Wateree
Ridgeway, SC

AU GRATIN POTATOES

- 4 medium potatoes
- 1 (5-ounce) can evaporated milk
- 1 (10¾-ounce) can cream of mushroom soup
- 1½ cups grated mild Cheddar cheese

Scrub and slice potatoes thin. Mix milk, soup and cheese until well blended. Layer potatoes and soup mixture in 8-inch square microwave dish. Cook in microwave for 18 minutes or until potatoes are tender.

Martha A. McCaghren
Enon Baptist Church
Danville, AL

GREEK POTATOES

Select amount of baking potatoes you desire. Boil until done; peel skin and quarter. Season with Greek seasoning, basil leaves and oregano. Heat skillet; add ¼ cup olive oil. Fry quartered, seasoned potatoes until all sides are golden brown.

George H. Johnson
Columbus Air Force Base Chapel
Columbus, MS

SWEET AND SOUR CARROTS

1 pound carrots, scraped and sliced
1 medium green pepper, chopped
⅓ cup sugar
1 teaspoon cornstarch
½ teaspoon salt
2 teaspoons soy sauce
1 teaspoon vinegar
1 (8-ounce) can pineapple chunks

Cook carrots in boiling water until tender. Add pepper; cook 3 minutes, drain and set aside. Combine sugar, cornstarch and salt, drain pineapple and reserve juice. Add enough water to juice to make ⅓ cup liquid; stir into sugar and cornstarch; add vinegar and soy sauce; cook over low heat until bubbly, stirring constantly. Stir in vegetables and pineapple, cook until well heated.

6-8 servings

Margaret T. Swindol
Booneville, MS

ONE SKILLET VEGGIE DELIGHT

2 large potatoes, peeled
1 large stick (not stalk) celery, diagonally sliced
2 large carrots, diagonally sliced
1 sweet potato
2 big onions (one yellow and one white)
½ head cabbage (red or green)
1 teaspoon pepper
Salt, to taste
¼ cup virgin olive oil
¾ cup water

Slice vegetables in order given into a large skillet that has a fitted lid. Sprinkle top with salt and pepper. Drizzle olive oil over top of veggie layers. Pour water over top. Cook on medium heat until cabbage is tender, not limp.

Serve with hot cornbread. Also great served with fresh salsa topping.

Shirlie Jensen
Prattville, AL

VEGGIE BARS

- 1 (8-ounce) package crescent rolls
- 1 cup broccoli, chopped
- 1 cup cauliflower, chopped
- 1 cup mild Cheddar cheese, shredded
- 1 cup carrots, shredded
- 1 (8-ounce) carton sour cream
- 1 (8-ounce) package cream cheese
- 1 cup Miracle Whip
- 1 (1-ounce) package dry ranch dressing mix

Line bottom of 9 x 13 inch baking dish or pan with rolls. Cook at 350° for 10 to 15 minutes until done. Let cool. Mix together cream cheese, sour cream, Miracle Whip and dressing mix with mixer until smooth and spread over rolls. Mix together all vegetables and layer on top of spread. Sprinkle shredded cheese on top. Cover with plastic wrap and press down to set vegetables. Refrigerate, preferably overnight or at least several hours. Cut in squares to serve.

24 squares

Jean Hood
Santa Fe Baptist Church
Santa Fe, TN

BEAN BAKE

- 1 (15.8-ounce) can great Northern beans, undrained
- ¼ teaspoon salt
- ¼ teaspoon prepared mustard
- 1½ tablespoons brown sugar
- ⅓ cup tomato juice
- 2 tablespoons chopped onion

Combine all ingredients. Bake in small greased casserole dish 30 to 40 minutes at 400°.

Nancy Davis
Parkwood Baptist Church
Concord, NC

CREAMED GREEN BEANS

- 3 tablespoons butter, divided
- ½ cup crushed cornflakes
- 1 tablespoon all-purpose flour
- ¼ teaspoon salt
- ¼ teaspoon pepper
- 1 teaspoon dried minced onion
- 1 teaspoon sugar
- 1 cup sour cream
- 4-6 cups French style green beans, cooked and drained
- 1 cup sharp Cheddar cheese, shredded

In small saucepan melt 1 tablespoon butter, stir in cornflake crumbs and set aside. Melt remaining butter in large saucepan. Stir in flour, salt, pepper, onion and sugar; heat and stir until bubbly. Reduce heat; add sour cream and stir until smooth. Cook and stir over low heat for 2 minutes (do not boil) Fold in beans. Spread into greased 1½-quart baking dish. Sprinkle cheese evenly over this and top with cornflake mixture. Bake uncovered at 400° for 20 minutes.

Serves 6-8

Irene Smith
Chiefland, FL

ITALIAN GREEN BEANS

- 3 (14½-ounce) cans green beans
- 1 (10-ounce) can tomatoes with green chiles
- 1 large onion, chopped
- 3-4 slices bacon
- Creole seasoning mix, to taste

Sauté onion and bacon. Add drained beans and tomatoes with chiles. Cover and simmer 35 to 45 minutes. Add seasoning to taste.

Doris McCauley
Woodland Baptist
Beaumont, Texas

LENTIL STROGANOFF

1 (16-ounce) bag dry lentils
3 cups water
11 vegetable bouillon cubes
2 bay leaves
1-2 cloves garlic
⅓ cup cocktail sherry
½ cup chopped onion
½ cup chopped red bell pepper
2 cups sliced, fresh mushrooms
1 cup low fat sour cream
Non-stick cooking spray

Sort through lentils, rinse and drain. Place lentils in 2-quart saucepan and cover with 3 cups water, plus bay leaves and garlic. Bring to a boil, reduce to simmer, cover with a lid and cook for 45 minutes. Meanwhile, sauté onions, bell pepper and mushrooms in pan with non-stick spray until lightly browned. Remove bay leaves from cooked lentils and add the vegetables and sherry. Just before serving stir in 1 cup sour cream, blend well and serve over noodles or rice.

Alice Lawrence
Stetson Baptist Church
Deland, FL

EGGPLANT AND MUSHROOMS

1 large eggplant
½ pound fresh mushrooms, sliced
1 (10-ounce) package seasoning blend
4 ounces butter
½ teaspoon Creole seasoning

Peel eggplant, cut in chunks and put in microwave pan. Cover and cook in microwave about 8 to 10 minutes until tender. Meanwhile melt butter and sauté seasoning blend and mushrooms until clear and dry. Add eggplant and seasoning. Cook on low about 5 minutes.

Marjorie Kieffer
Sulphur, LA

SCALLOPED TOMATOES AND CHEESE

- 1 (28-ounce) can tomatoes
- 2 teaspoons sugar
- 1½ cups soft bread crumbs
- ¼ cup melted butter
- 1 cup grated American cheese
- Salt and pepper, to taste

Season tomatoes to taste with salt and pepper. Add sugar, combine crumbs and melted butter. Arrange layers of tomatoes, cheese and crumbs in casserole, ending with crumbs. Bake at 350° for 15 to 20 minutes.

6 servings

Betty Baker
First Baptist Church
Westminster, SC

TOMATO PIE

- 1 unbaked deep dish pie shell
- 2-3 tomatoes, peeled and sliced
- 1 large onion, sliced thinly
- 2 cups shredded sharp Cheddar cheese
- 3 tablespoons mayonnaise
- Seasonings and spices, to taste

Partially bake pie shell. Layer onions, then tomatoes and sprinkle with salt, pepper and spices. Repeat layers until all tomatoes and onions are used. Mix cheese and mayonnaise and spread over the top layer. Bake at 350° for 30 minutes or longer.

Paula Suddreth
Pleasant Garden Baptist Church
Greensboro, NC

TOMATO PIE

12 slices bacon, cooked
3 large tomatoes, sliced
1 (8-inch) deep dish pie crust, baked
8 green spring onions, chopped
1 cup grated Cheddar cheese
1 cup mayonnaise (can reduce to ½ cup)

In baked pie shell arrange tomatoes and onions, crumble bacon on top. Mix grated cheese and mayonnaise; spread on top of pie. Bake at 350° for 30 minutes.

Dorothy Culbreth
Dothan, AL

ZITA BAKE

1 (8-ounce) package Zita noodles
1 (24-ounce) jar fat-free spaghetti sauce
1 (12-ounce) carton non-fat cottage cheese
2 cups grated fat-free mozzarella cheese

Cook noodles in boiling water until tender. Drain, layer noodles with cottage cheese and spaghetti sauce in a baking dish. Sprinkle mozzarella cheese on top. Bake at 350° about 20 to 25 minutes until bubbly.

Ginny Brooks
Parkwood Baptist Church
Concord, NC

DIRTY RICE

- 1 stick butter, melted
- 1 cup rice
- ½ cup chopped bell pepper
- ½ cup chopped onion
- 1 (8-ounce) can mushroom pieces
- 1 (10¾-ounce) can cream of mushroom soup
- 1 (10½-ounce) can beef consommé

Melt butter in medium to large casserole dish. Add rice, then sprinkle pepper, onion, mushroom, using juice from mushrooms. Add enough water to fill the soup can. Mix water and soups and warm slowly. Pour over rice mixture and cook 30 minutes at 350° or until mushrooms come to top.

Serve with a fresh green salad and you have a meal.

Sarah Shiver
Pathway Baptist Church
Dothan, AL

DIRTY RICE

- 1 cup rice (uncooked)
- 1 medium onion, chopped
- ½ stick butter
- 1 (10½-ounce) can beef consommé or beef broth
- 1 (10¾-ounce) can cream of mushroom soup
- 1 (8-ounce) can mushrooms with juice
- 1 cup water if desired

Brown onion in butter. Mix with other ingredients and pour into 9 x 13 inch baking dish, cover and cook 1 hour at 350°.

Rhonda Johnson
Bethel Baptist Church
Dothan, AL

GERMAN SWEET RICE

- 1 cup raw rice
- 2½ cups water
- 1 (12-ounce) can evaporated milk
- ¾ cup sugar
- Pinch of salt
- Sugar and cinnamon, to taste

Cover rice with water; add salt and cook until almost soft, adding water as needed. Add can of milk and sugar. Cook until rice is soft, but still thin. It will thicken as it cools. Pour into glass dish and sprinkle with sugar and cinnamon.

Best when served warm

Joyce Dossey
Gassville Baptist Church
Cotter, AR

HOT RICE

- 1 pound hot sausage
- 1 bell pepper, diced
- 1 onion, diced
- 1 cup Minute Rice
- 2 (2.1-ounce) envelopes dry chicken noodle soup
- 5 cups water
- 1 (8-ounce) package processed cheese product

Cook sausage, bell pepper and onion; boil water add Minute Rice and cook for 10 minutes then add dry noodle soup, cook for 10 minutes, add sausage, pepper and onion mix. Add processed cheese product, and pour into 9 x 13 inch casserole dish. Bake in 350° oven until bubbly.

Fay Hatcher
Columbus Air Force Base Chapel
Columbus, MS

CAJUN RICE AND SAUSAGE

- 1 (8-ounce) package smoked sausage, sliced in ½-inch pieces
- 1 large onion, chopped
- 1 large bell pepper, diced
- ½ cup diced celery
- 1 (4.5-ounce) package Cajun style rice and sauce
- 4 cups water

Brown sausage and onion; add bell pepper and cook for 3 minutes. Stir in celery, rice mix, and water; bring to a boil. Reduce heat and cover; simmer, stirring occasionally until rice is tender (about 10 minutes).

Rudy Branham
Sawney's Creek Baptist Church
Elgin, SC

POTATOES AND HAM AU GRATIN

- ⅓ cup chopped green onions
- 1 clove minced garlic
- 2 tablespoons butter
- 1½ cups light cream or half-and-half
- ⅓ cup spicy mustard
- ⅔ cup shredded Cheddar cheese, divided
- 2 tablespoons chopped parsley, divided
- 6 medium potatoes, thinly sliced
- 1½ cups cooked ham, diced

Cook and stir onions and garlic in butter in medium saucepan until tender. Reduce heat to low and stir in cream, mustard and ⅓ cup Cheddar cheese. Cook and stir until cheese melts and mixture is smooth. Add 1 tablespoon parsley and layer ⅓ of potatoes, ham and cream sauce in greased 9-inch square baking dish. Repeat layers twice, ending with cream cheese sauce. Sprinkle top with remaining cheese. Cover with foil. Bake at 375° for 45 minutes, remove foil and bake 15 to 20 minutes more until tender. Let stand 5 minutes. Garnish with remaining parsley.

Alice Rickman
Pinewood Baptist Church
Pinewood, SC

MARINATED CUCUMBERS

1 cup water
½ cup sugar
½ cup vinegar
1 teaspoon celery seeds
3-4 cucumbers, sliced
2 large onions, sliced

Heat water, sugar, vinegar and celery seeds until sugar is dissolved. Let cool. Pour this liquid over cucumbers and onions and refrigerate overnight.

Roberta Johnson-Ford
Madisonville, KY

CHOW CHOW

1 gallon green tomatoes
1 gallon red and green bell peppers, mixed
1 gallon onions
2 medium cabbages
5 pounds sugar
½ gallon hot pepper
½ cup salt

Chop all ingredients. Wear gloves if you cut up the hot pepper by hand, so you don't blister your hands. Cover all ingredients with vinegar. Bring to a boil and boil for 25 minutes. Put in canning jars.

Susan B. Fowler
Clear Spring Baptist Church
Simpsonville, SC

Casseroles

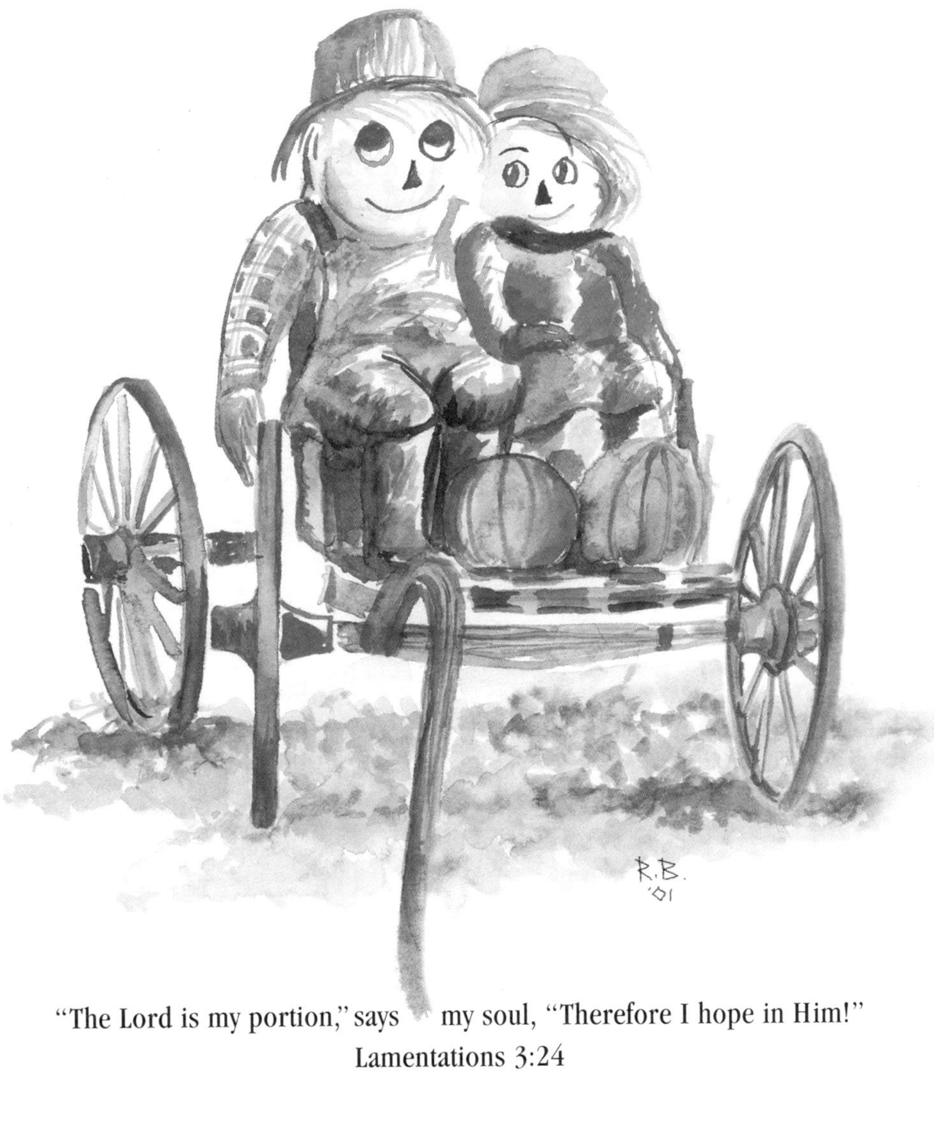

"The Lord is my portion," says my soul, "Therefore I hope in Him!"
Lamentations 3:24

APPLE CHEESE CASSEROLE

2 (16-ounce) cans sliced apples
1 stick of margarine
1 cup sugar
¾ cup flour (self-rising)
1 (8-ounce) package processed cheese loaf

Place the apples in a 9 x 13 inch dish. Add the margarine, flour, sugar, and cheese in a boiler. Cook until creamy. Pour over apples. Bake 30 to 40 minutes at 350°.

Edna Earl Lawrence
First Baptist Church,
Vernon, AL

HOT PINEAPPLE CASSEROLE

¾ cup sugar
5 tablespoons flour
2 (15¼-ounce) cans chuck pineapple, drained
1½ cups grated Cheddar cheese
1 stick margarine, melted
1 tube Ritz crackers, crushed

Mix sugar and flour. Layer drained pineapple in 13 x 9 inch pan or baking dish. Sprinkle sugar mixture over pineapple. Next, sprinkle cheese evenly over pineapple/flour mixture. Spread Ritz cracker crumbs over top. Pour melted margarine over top. Bake at 350° for 25 minutes.

This is delicious with ham, chicken, or any main dish.

Mildred L. Henry
Gainesville GA

TURNIP CASSEROLE

5 small turnips
2 tablespoons margarine
1½ cups milk
½ cup shredded Cheddar cheese
1 cup soft bread crumbs
½ teaspoon salt
⅛ teaspoon pepper
½ cup soft bread crumbs
1 tablespoon margarine, melted

Cook turnips and set aside. Melt 2 tablespoons margarine; stir in milk. Add bread crumbs, cheese, salt and pepper. Cook over low heat, stirring until thickened. Stir in turnips. Spoon mixture into 1½-quart greased casserole dish. Combine ½ cup breadcrumbs and 1 tablespoon margarine, sprinkle over casserole and bake for 20 minutes at 350°.

6-8 servings

Genevieve Hagy
Harlan KY

CARROT CASSEROLE

1 pound carrots
1 cup mayonnaise
2 tablespoons prepared horseradish
2 tablespoons grated onion
1 tube round, buttery crackers
1-2 tablespoons butter

Wash, scrape and slice carrots. Cook in water until tender. Drain well and mix with next 3 ingredients. Place in casserole and top with crushed Ritz crackers mixed with small amount of butter. Bake 325° to 350° about 15 minutes until top is lightly browned

Mary Ann Ballard
Holly Grove Baptist Church
Brownsville, TN

HOMINY CASSEROLE

- 1 onion, chopped
- 1 stick margarine
- 2 (15½-ounce) cans of yellow or white hominy, drained
- ½ cup water
- 1 (10¾-ounce) can mushroom soup
- 1 (8-ounce) jar cheese spread
- 1 (10½-ounce) corn chips

Combine the above ingredients except corn chips. Place in a casserole dish. Cover with crushed corn chips. Bake at 375° until bubbly.

Judy Morisset
First Baptist Church
Ozark, MO

VIDALIA ONION CASSEROLE

- 4-5 big onions, cut in ½-inch slices
- 1 stick margarine
- 3 ounces or more grated Cheddar cheese
- 1½ stacks round, buttery crackers, crushed

Separate onion into rings. Cook onions in microwave with margarine until limp. Layer onions, crackers, cheese and margarine in 9 x 13 inch casserole dish. Bake at 350° for about 25 minutes.

Verlon Honeycutt
First Baptist Church
Booneville, MS

HOT DOG CASSEROLE

- 8 wieners
- 1 tablespoon butter
- 1 (8-ounce) can tomato sauce
- ½ teaspoon garlic salt
- 1 teaspoon sugar
- 2 cups cooked noodles
- 1 (3-ounce) package cream cheese
- ½ cup sour cream
- ½ cup grated Cheddar cheese

Melt butter in skillet and heat wieners which have been cut into ½-inch chunks. Add tomato sauce, garlic salt and sugar; heat. Place noodles in a greased 9 x 13 inch casserole dish. Mix cream cheese and sour cream with fork. Spoon over noodles. Add wieners and tomato sauce. Sprinkle top with grated cheese and bake at 350° for 30 minutes.

Linda Vaughn
Mt. Beulah Baptist
Morven, NC

PORK CHOP CASSEROLE

- 2 (14½-ounce) cans French style green beans, drained
- 1 box Pork Stove Top Dressing
- 4 nice size pork chops

In 9 x 13 inch baking dish, cover bottom of dish with both cans of green beans. Mix stove top dressing, uncooked and on the moist side. Spread on top of green beans. Lay pork chops on top of dressing. Bake at 375° for 45 minutes or until pork chops are crispy.

Tommy Painter
First Baptist Church
Boiling Springs,SC

CHEESY HAM CASSEROLE

- ½ cup salad dressing
- 2 cups fresh or frozen broccoli florets
- 1½ cups (6-ounce) shredded sharp cheese
- 1½ cups chopped ham
- 1½ cups corkscrew noodles
- ½ cup chopped red or green bell peppers
- ¼ cup milk
- ¾ cup seasoned croutons (optional)
- ¼ cup chopped onion (optional)
- 1 garlic clove (optional)

If using fresh broccoli, blanch in hot water for one minute, drain and let cool for about five minutes. Cook corkscrew noodles according to package directions. Mix all ingredients except ½ cup cheese and croutons. Spoon into a 1½-quart casserole dish. Sprinkle with remaining cheese. Bake at 350° for 20 minutes then top with croutons for the last 10 minutes.

I like this as a pasta salad rather than baked.

LaRue McDaniel
Glen Hope Baptist Church
Burlington, NC

PLANTATION LAYERED CASSEROLE

- 2½ cups crispy rice cereal (saving ½ cup for top)
- 1 pound bulk sausage
- 1 small onion, chopped
- 1 cup rice, cooked
- 10 ounces grated sharp cheese
- 3 eggs
- 1 (10¾-ounce) can mushroom soup
- ¼ cup milk

Sauté sausage and onion. Combine with 2 cups rice cereal, rice and cheese and place in a 2-quart casserole dish. Combine eggs, soup and milk. Pour over mixture; punch holes to penetrate. Top with remaining ½ cup rice cereal and refrigerate overnight. Bake at 350° for 30 minutes.

Grace A. Tarrant
The Chapel at Lake Wateree
Ridgeway, SC

HAWAIIAN SAUSAGE CASSEROLE

1 (20-ounce) can chunk pineapple
1 (16-ounce) can sweet potatoes, cut into ½-inch chunks
¾ pound smoked sausage, cut into ½-inch chunks
3 tablespoons brown sugar
2 tablespoons cornstarch
¼ teaspoon salt
1 tablespoon butter

Drain pineapple and potatoes, reserving 1¼ cups juice. Set aside. Place pineapple, potatoes, and sausage in a 10 x 6 x 2 inch baking dish. Set aside. Combine sugar, cornstarch and salt in a saucepan. Gradually add pineapple/potato juice mixture, stirring until blended. Cook, stirring constantly, until mixture thickens, and comes to a boil. Boil 1 minute, stirring constantly. Remove from heat and add butter. Pour over mixture in baking dish. Cover and bake at 350° for 35 minutes.

Ralph N. Brown
First Baptist Church
Lucedale, MS

ZUCCHINI CASSEROLE

6 cups cubed zucchini
1 cup shredded carrot
½ cup finely chopped onion
1 (10¾-ounce) can cream of chicken soup
1 cup sour cream
1 (8-ounce) package herbed stuffing
½ cup margarine, melted

Cook zucchini, carrots and onion for 5 minutes. Mix chicken soup and sour cream together and combine with vegetables. Mix stuffing crumbs and melted margarine. Put ½ cup crumb mixture in bottom of large, shallow pan. Add zucchini mixture; top with rema[illegible] at 350° for 30 minutes or until crumbs are brown[illegible] almost bubbly.

College He[illegible]

YELLOW CROOKNECK SQUASH CASSEROLE

- 6 yellow crookneck squash
- 1 pound hot bulk sausage
- 4 medium onions, diced
- 1 cup diced celery
- 2 cloves garlic
- 4 slices toasted bread
- 1 cup sharp Cheddar cheese
- 1 cup water

Optional seasonings of Parmesan cheese, oregano, sage, cumin , Italian bread crumbs and red pepper

Boil squash in salted water until tender; drain. Sauté sausage, celery, onion and garlic until brown. Add 1 cup water and boil until tender Add squash, crumbled toast, Cheddar cheese, oregano, sage, cumin and red pepper to taste. Pour mixture into greased covered casserole. Top with Parmesan cheese and dust with Italian bread crumbs. Cover and cook at 350° for 30 minutes. Remove cover 10 minutes before serving.

Esther L. Keane
First Baptist Church
Vernon, AL

SQUASH CASSEROLE

- 2½ pounds yellow squash
- 1 (8-ounce) carton sour cream
- 1 (10¾-ounce) can cream of chicken soup
- 2 carrots, grated
- 2 medium onions, chopped
- 2 teaspoons black pepper

Wash and cut up squash and boil until tender. Drain well. Mix above ingredients.

- 1 (8-ounce) package herb seasoned Pepperidge Farm dressing mix
- 2 sticks margarine

Melt margarine in sauce pan. Add dressing mix and stir until mix is coated with oleo. Butter 9 x 13 inch casserole dish. Pour in squash mixture and put dressing mix and butter on top. Pat Down. Bake at 350° for 45 minutes.

Doll Peterson
First Baptist Church
Bay Minette, AL

HASH BROWN CASSEROLE

- 1 (2-pound) bag frozen, shredded hash browns
- 1 stick margarine
- 1 (10¾-ounce) can cream of chicken soup
- ½ cup chopped onion
- 2 cups sour cream
- 1 teaspoon salt
- 1 teaspoon pepper

Thaw potatoes; mix all ingredients thoroughly. Spread in 9 x 13 inch, well buttered glass baking dish.

- 2 cups cornflakes
- ¼ cup margarine
- 1¼ cups shredded sharp cheese

Crush cornflakes. Add margarine. Spread over casserole. Bake at 350° for 35 minutes. Remove from oven. Spread cheese over cornflakes. Return to oven for 5 minutes.

Margaret Colvin
Sawney's Creek Church
Lugoff, S.C.

IRISH POTATO CASSEROLE

- 6 medium potatoes
- ½ cup butter
- 1 (10¾-ounce) can cream of chicken soup
- 1½ cups grated cheese
- 3 tablespoons minced onion
- 1 (8-ounce) carton sour cream
- 1 teaspoon salt
- 1 cup cornflakes
- 1 tablespoon butter

Boil potatoes in peeling 15 or 20 minutes. Peel and grate. Then heat soup and ½ cup butter; add cheese, onion, sour cream and salt. Mix with potatoes and pour into 9 x 13 inch baking dish. Melt 1 tablespoon butter and pour over crushed cornflakes which have been spread on top of casserole. Bake 350° for 45 to 60 minutes

Estelle Barnett
Locust Hill Baptist Church,
Travelers Rest, SC

POTATO CASSEROLE

- 8-10 potatoes, sliced and parboiled
- 1 pound processed cheese loaf
- 1 stick butter
- ½ cup green onion
- 1 (10¾-ounce) can cream of chicken soup
- 1 (8-ounce) carton sour cream
- 1 (3-ounce) jar bacon bits

Melt cheese loaf and butter. Add green onions, chicken soup and sour cream. Pour potatoes into casserole dish; cover with cheese sauce. Top with one bottle real bacon bits. Bake 350° until bubbly.

Yvonne H. Vining
First Baptist Church
Amite, LA

RICE CASSEROLE

- 1 cup regular rice, uncooked
- 1 (10½-ounce) can beef broth
- 1 (10¾-ounce) can French onion soup
- 1 (4½-ounce) jar sliced mushrooms, drained
- 1 stick butter

Melt butter and mix all other ingredients together. Put in 9 x 13 inch baking dish. Cook 350° for 35 to 40 minutes.

Glyneice Lovvorn,
Bowden, GA

RICE AND CORN CASSEROLE

1 (5-ounce) package yellow rice
1 (11-ounce) can Niblet's Mexicorn
1 (10¾-ounce) can cream of chicken soup
1 cup grated Cheddar cheese

Cook rice. Add corn and soup. Put in 9 x 13 inch casserole dish and top with grated cheese. Bake 350° for 15 to 20 minutes.

Becky May
Macedonia Baptist Church
Mendenhall, MS

VEG-ALL CASSEROLE

2 (15-ounce) cans Veg-All
1 (8-ounce) can water chestnuts, drained
1 cup chopped celery
1 cup sharp Cheddar cheese, grated
1 onion, diced
¾ cup mayonnaise
½ stick margarine

Sauté onion and celery in butter until tender. Add to remaining ingredients and mix well. Put in 9 x 13 inch casserole dish and bake at 350° for 30 minutes.

Betty R. Noler
Lincoln, NC

...IXED VEGETABLE CASSEROLE

2 (1... ...ce) packages frozen mixed vegetables
1 (8-ounce) can water chestnuts, drained and diced
1 medium onion, chopped
1½ cups Hellmann's mayonnaise
1½ cups grated cheese
1½ cups round, buttery cracker crumbs
½ stick butter
Paprika

Cook vegetables as directed on package. Drain. Mix vegetables, onion, water chestnuts, and mayonnaise. Put into greased casserole. Top with grated cheese. Mix cracker crumbs with ½ stick melted margarine and sprinkle on top. Sprinkle top with paprika. Bake until lightly brown at 350°

I sprinkle a little paprika and black pepper in the vegetable mixture.

Clara Belle Jewell
Hillside Baptist Church

FRENCH BEAN AND CORN CASSEROLE

1 (14½-ounce) can French style green beans, drained
1 (11-ounce) can whole kernel corn, drained
1 medium onion, chopped
½ cup grated cheese
1 (10¾-ounce) can cream of celery soup
1 (8-ounce) carton sour cream
1 stick margarine
1 stack round, buttery crackers

Mix beans and corn; put in ungreased 9 x 13 inch casserole dish. Mix soup, sour cream, cheese, onion and salt; spread on beans and corn. Mix margarine with crackers and put on top of mixture. Bake in 350° oven for 35 minutes

Mildred Williams
Second Baptist Church,
Warner Robins, GA

BEAN CASSEROLE

- 1 pound hamburger
- 1 medium onion
- 1 cup catsup
- ½ teaspoon dried mustard
- ½ cup brown sugar
- 2 teaspoons Worcestershire sauce
- ½ cup water
- 2 teaspoons chili powder
- 1 (23-ounce) can pork and beans

Brown hamburger and onion and drain. Add remaining ingredients except for pork and beans and simmer 20 minutes, add pork and beans. Cook 5 to 10 minutes and serve.

Dorothy Culbreth
Dothan AL

SWEET POTATO CASSEROLE

- 3 cups sweet potatoes (about 4 large ones)
- ½ cup sugar
- 2 eggs, beaten
- ⅓ cup milk
- ½ cup butter
- 1 teaspoon vanilla

Boil and mash potatoes. Mix in sugar, butter, eggs, vanilla and milk. Place in 9 x 13 inch casserole dish.

- ⅓ cup melted butter
- ½ cup flour
- 1 cup light brown sugar
- 1 cup chopped pecans

Melt butter and add remaining ingredients; sprinkle on top of potatoes. Bake in 350° oven for 25 minutes.

Ruth Hagler
Broaddus, TX

CHICKEN AND DRESSING CASSEROLE

- 8 chicken breasts or 1 whole chicken
- 2 tablespoons butter or margarine
- 2 (10¾-ounce) cans cream of chicken soup
- ¾ cup milk
- 2¼ cups chicken broth
- 1 (8-ounce) bag herb deasoned Pepperidge Farm dressing mix
- 1½ stalks celery, chopped
- 1 small onion, chopped
- 1 egg, beaten

Boil chicken until tender; salt to taste. Cool and remove skin and bones. Place chicken in long baking dish. Add pepper to taste and dot with butter or margarine. (Save chicken broth.) Mix cream of chicken soup, ¼ cup chicken broth and milk. Pour this over chicken. Sauté celery and onions in butter or margarine. Add this to dressing mix, beaten egg and 1½ cups chicken broth. Spread over chicken and soup. Bake 350° for 45 minutes covered. Uncover and bake 15 minutes longer.

Patsy E. Dinkins
Sawney's Creek Baptist Church,
Ridgeway, SC

6 CAN CASSEROLE

- 1 (10¾-ounce) can cream of chicken soup
- 1 (10¾-ounce) can cream of mushroom soup
- 1 (4½-ounce) jar mushrooms, drained
- 1 (8-ounce) can water chestnuts, sliced and drained
- 1 (5-ounce) can evaporated milk
- 1 small can Chinese noodles
- 2 cups cooked chicken, diced
- Parmesan cheese

Mix all ingredients. Place in 9 x 13 inch casserole dish and top with Parmesan cheese. Bake at 350° for 30 minutes.

Elaine Fuller
Westwood Baptist Church,
Birmingham, AL

POPPY SEED CHICKEN

- 6-8 chicken breasts, cooked, boned, chopped
- 1 (10¾-ounce) can cream of celery soup
- 1 (2¼-ounce) package slivered almonds
- 1 (10¾-ounce) can cream of mushroom soup
- 1 cup sour cream

Mix the above and spread in a buttered 9 x 13 inch casserole dish.

- 1 stick margarine, melted
- 1 package club crackers (⅓ of a box)
- 2-3 tablespoons poppy seed

Mix the above and spread over chicken mixture. Bake 20 to 30 minutes in 350° oven (or until hot in middle).

LaRue McDaniel
Glen Hope Baptist Church
Burlington, NC

QUICK CHICKEN CASSEROLE

- 4 large chicken breasts
- 1 (8-ounce) carton sour cream
- 1 (10¾-ounce) can cream of chicken soup
- 1 stick butter
- 1 tube round, buttery crackers

Boil and debone chicken; tear into small pieces and line bottom of 9 x 13 inch casserole dish. Mix together soup and sour cream; heat just to boiling, stir well and pour over chicken. Crumble all crackers over mixture. Melt butter and spread over crackers. Bake at 350° for 20 minutes.

Jean Hood
Santa Fe Baptist Church
Santa Fe, TN

DORITOS, CHICKEN & CHEESE CASSEROLE

- 2-3 pounds chicken breasts
- 2 medium onions, chopped
- 2 (10¾-ounce) cans cream of chicken soup
- 1 can water
- 4-5 small, pickled jalapeño peppers, chopped
- 1 (9-ounce) jar Cheez-Whiz
- 1 medium bag nacho flavored Doritos
- 1 medium bag taco flavored Doritos

Boil and debone chicken; cut into bite size. Mix onion, soup, water and peppers in saucepan. Cook over medium heat 25 minutes, stirring frequently. Add chicken and cook 6 minutes more. Crumble chips and line large casserole with ½ crumbled chips. Add chicken and cheese mixture and remaining chips. Bake at 300° for 20 to 25 minutes.

Janie Brooks
Lake Catoma Baptist Church
Cullman, AL

POPPY SEED CHICKEN

- 6 chicken breasts, cooked and cut into small pieces
- 1 (10¾-ounce) can cream of mushroom soup
- 1 (10¾-ounce) can cream of chicken soup
- 1 (16-ounce) carton sour cream
- 2 teaspoons poppy seed

Mix all these ingredients together and pour into 9 x 13 inch baking dish.

- 2 stacks round, buttery crackers
- 1½ sticks margarine

Crush crackers, melt margarine and pour over crackers. Spread cracker and margarine mix over chicken. Bake in 350° oven until hot and bubbly.

Serve over cooked rice.

Peggy Jones Krupski
Precision Valley Baptist Church
Springfield, VT

CHICKEN RICE-A-RONI CASSEROLE

5-6 chicken breasts
1 (10¾-ounce) can cream of chicken soup
1 (10¾-ounce) can chicken broth
1 stick margarine
1 box chicken Rice-A-Roni

Place uncooked chicken breasts in bottom of casserole dish. Mix all other ingredients and pour over top of chicken. Bake in 350° oven for 1 hour.

Fredia Longenecker
Rices Creek Baptist
Liberty, SC

CHICKEN CASSEROLE

1 cup cooked chicken
1 cup cooked rice
¼ cup slivered almonds
1 small onion, cut fine
1 teaspoon salt
½ cup mayonnaise
1 teaspoon lemon juice
¾ cup diced celery
2 hard-cooked eggs, cut up
1 (8-ounce) can mushrooms
1 (10¾-ounce) can undiluted mushroom soup
Crushed potato chips

Combine all but the potato chips in 9 x 13 inch casserole dish. Put in refrigerator overnight. Remove from refrigerator. Before cooking, sprinkle top with potato chips and cook uncovered at 375° for 30 minutes.

Vernon Chevallier
Sulphur, LA

CHICKEN RO-TEL

- 4 chicken breasts
- 1 (10-ounce) can Rotel tomatoes and green chiles
- 1 (16-ounce) package processed cheese loaf
- 1 (15-ounce) can English peas
- 1 green pepper, chopped
- 1 onion, chopped
- 1 stick margarine
- 1 (7-ounce) package spaghetti (break about 4 times)

Boil chicken breasts until cooked (reserve broth). Cool and chop. Cook spaghetti in chicken broth until tender Do not drain. Add cheese to spaghetti and let melt. Sauté onion and pepper in oleo until tender. Add peas, chicken and Rotel tomatoes. Mix all ingredients together and put in 9 x 13 inch casserole dish and bake at 350° for 35 minutes until liquid is absorbed.

When I boil my chicken, I put enough water to cover. It's best not to put too much water, you can always add more.

June Vines

HAMBURGER TATER TOT CASSEROLE

- 1½ pounds lean ground beef
- 1 (15-ounce) package frozen tater tots
- ¼ cup chopped onion
- 1 (10¾-ounce) can cream of mushroom soup

Crumble and cook beef until no longer pink. Don't overcook. Drain well. Press into 9 x 13 inch casserole dish. Sprinkle with onions; add tater tots. Pour soup over top. Bake in preheated 350° oven for 1 hour.

Yvonne Sherrill
Mt. Hebron Baptist Church
Spruce Pine, AL

HAMBURGER CASSEROLE

- 2 pounds ground beef
- 1 cup chopped onion
- 1 (15-ounce) can sweet peas
- 1 (8-ounce) package fine noodles, cooked
- ¾ cup shredded cheese
- 1 (10¾-ounce) can cream of chicken soup
- 1 (10¾-ounce) can cream of mushroom soup
- 1 cup sour cream
- 3 sprigs chopped parsley
- 1 tablespoon sugar

Fry ground beef and onions. Drain. Add remaining ingredients. Place in 2-quart casserole and top with buttered bread crumbs and bake 350° for 1 hour.

Jane Johnson
Pine Forest Congregational Christian
Valley, AL

CRITTENDON CASSEROLE

- 1 (8-ounce) package egg noodles
- 1 (10¾-ounce) can cream of mushroom soup
- 1 soup can milk
- ½ pound grated sharp Cheddar cheese
- ¾ cup ripe olives, chopped
- 3 tablespoons parsley, chopped
- ½ cup onions, chopped
- 2 pounds lean ground beef
- 1 can Chinese noodles
- ¼ pound slivered blanched almonds
- Salt and pepper, to taste

Cook noodles, brown meat slightly in heavy skillet, add onions, salt and pepper and blend. Combine soup and milk and blend. In large casserole, put layer of noodles, cheese, olives, parsley, then meat. Repeat layers until all ingredients are used. Pour soup mixture over all and bake 350° for 35 to 40 minutes. Remove from oven; top with Chinese noodles and almonds. Bake 10 to 15 minutes longer.

If dry, add a little milk.

Linda Vaughn
Mt. Beulah Baptist Church
Morven, NC

BEEF-IN CASSEROLE

- 2½ pounds ground chuck
- 1 teaspoon garlic juice
- 4 tablespoons margarine
- 2 (8-ounce) cans tomato sauce
- 1 teaspoon sugar
- 1 (8-ounce) package cream cheese
- 1 (16-ounce) carton sour cream
- 1 cup grated cheese
- 4 green onions, tops and all
- 1 (10-ounce) package medium egg noodles
- 1 (10¾-ounce) can cream of mushroom soup
- Salt and pepper, to taste
- Margarine

Brown meat in margarine, drain, add garlic juice and simmer 20 minutes. Add tomato sauce, salt, pepper and sugar and simmer 15 minutes. In separate bowl mix cream cheese, sour cream and chopped onions. Set aside. Cook noodles. In large casserole or 2 smaller ones, layer noodles, meat, grated cheese, sour cream mixture, in that order until all used. Top with undiluted mushroom soup. Bake at 325° for 30 minutes or until hot and bubbly. Last 10 minutes sprinkle with extra Cheddar cheese.

Verlon Honeycutt
First Baptist Church
Booneville, MS

COMPANY CASSEROLE

- ¾ pound ground round
- 1 medium onion, chopped
- 2 cups canned tomatoes
- 1 tablespoon steak sauce
- 5 ounces macaroni, cooked
- ½ cup lowfat cheese
- 1 tablespoon catsup
- 1 (10¾-ounce) can 99% fat free cream of mushroom soup

Brown ground round and drain. Add onion, tomatoes, steak sauce and catsup. Simmer for 30 minutes. Add macaroni. Pour into 9-inch baking dish or pan. Top with soup and cheese. Bake for 30 minutes at 350°.

Sarah H. Hager
Troutman Baptist Church
Troutman, NC

CHEROKEE CASSEROLE (1950'S STYLE)

- 1 pound hamburger
- 1/8 teaspoon oregano
- 1/8 teaspoon thyme
- Garlic powder, to taste
- Salt and pepper, to taste
- 1 (10¾-ounce) can cream of mushroom soup
- 1 (14½-ounce) can whole tomatoes
- 1 cup Minute Rice
- Olives
- Pasteurized processed cheese

Brown hamburger meat and drain. Add other ingredients and simmer until thickened. Place in casserole dish and strip with cheese strips and pimento olives (making squares). Broil until cheese melts.

Makes a good main dish meal with salad.

Dorothy G. Bristow
Parkwood Church of God
Fort Wayne, IN

HAMBURGER CASSEROLE

- 1 pound hamburger
- 1 large onion, chopped
- ½ green pepper, chopped
- 1 clove minced garlic
- 1 teaspoon salt
- ½ teaspoon pepper
- 1 tablespoon chili powder
- 1 teaspoon sugar
- 2 (8-ounce) cans tomato sauce
- 1 (8-ounce) package noodles or shells
- Few shakes of hamburger seasoning

Brown hamburger, add onion, green pepper, garlic, tomato sauce and seasonings. Place noodles (cooked and buttered) into buttered casserole. Pour hamburger mixture over noodles. Add shredded cheese on top. Bake at 350° for 20 minutes.

Judy Morisset
First Baptist Church
Ozark, MO

SPAGHETTI CASSEROLE

1 pound ground round beef
2 medium onions, chopped
½ cup tomato juice
1 (8-ounce) box spaghetti
1 (8-ounce) can tomato sauce
½ can water
1 (4-ounce) can tomato paste
4 ounces water
2-3 cups grated sharp Cheddar cheese
1½ (10¾-ounce) cans mushroom soup
Sliced green olives

Break up meat and sauté in a saucepan with onion until meat loses all red color. Drain off any grease. Add tomato juice, tomato sauce, ½ can water, and tomato paste with can of water. Cover and let mixture come to a boil. Then reduce heat and simmer for 30 minutes. While this is cooking, break up spaghetti and cook in boiling, salted water according to box directions. When spaghetti is done, drain. Place into greased 9 x 13 inch casserole (or into two 8 x 8 inch casseroles). Add a layer of sauce, a layer of spaghetti and a layer of cheese. Repeat these layers until it is all used. Over the top layer add the mushroom soup and sliced olives. Bake for 30 minutes at 350° until bubbly.

Frances Tate
Parkwood Baptist Church
Concord, NC

CHICKEN IN ONION SOUP

3 cups water
½ stick butter
1 (1¼-ounce) envelope onion soup mix
1 whole chicken

Put water and butter in pan and bring to boil. Add onion soup mix and remove from heat. Let set while you prepare chicken (cut up, salt, pepper and flour). Place chicken in a 13 x 9 inch pan and pour soup over it. Bake uncovered about 1 hour in 350° oven. Make gravy from soup mixture.

Carolyn Mace
Amboy Baptist Church
North Little Rock, AR

CHRISTY'S CASSEROLE

1 (8-ounce) package cream cheese
2 cups sour cream
1 teaspoon salt
½ teaspoon pepper
3 medium onions, diced
1½ pounds ground beef
2 tablespoons butter
2 (8-ounce) cans tomato sauce
1 tablespoon sugar
1 teaspoon Worcestershire sauce
2 (5-ounce) packages thin egg noodles
½ cup shredded Cheddar cheese

Mix cream cheese, sour cream, salt, pepper and onions. Set aside. Brown beef in butter; add tomato sauce, sugar and Worcestershire sauce. Cook noodles as directed on package. Spread ½ noodles, ½ meat mixture and ½ cheese mixture in casserole dish. Repeat this process. Top with Cheddar cheese. Bake at 350° for 30 minutes.

Linda Vaughn
Mt. Beulah Baptist Church
Morven, NC

MEXICAN CORNBREAD CASSEROLE

1½ pounds ground beef
1 small onion, diced
1 small bell pepper, chopped
1 teaspoon garlic
1 teaspoon red pepper
Salt and pepper, to taste
1 (15-ounce) can green peas
1 (15¼-ounce) can whole kernel corn
1 (8½-ounce) package Mexican cornbread mix
1 cup grated Cheddar cheese

Brown ground beef; drain and sauté onion, pepper, garlic and pepper until veggies are done. Add green peas and corn and pour into 9 x 13 inch dish sprayed with non-stick cooking spray. Top with dry cornbread mix and Cheddar cheese. Bake at 350° for 30 minutes.

Serve with green salad and your meal is complete

Juanita Blackwell
Maplewood First Baptist Church
Sulphur, LA

ENCHILADA CASSEROLE

- 2 pounds ground meat
- 1 can enchilada sauce (mild)
- Salt and pepper, to taste
- 1 package frozen tortillas (12 corn)
- Garlic powder, to taste
- 1 pound processed cheese loaf
- 1 (10-ounce) can tomatoes and green chiles
- 2 (10¾-ounce) cans mushroom soup

Add garlic powder, salt and pepper to ground meat and brown. Drain and add enchilada sauce and put in greased 9 x 13 inch pan. Alternate layers of tortillas and cheese over meat. Put tomatoes and chiles over this. Heat mushroom soup and spread over top. Bake 1 hour at 350° uncovered.

Carolyn Mace
Amboy Baptist Church
North Little Rock, AR

MEXICAN CORN CASSEROLE

- 2 (14¾-ounce) cans cream corn
- 1 (8½-ounce) package jalapeño cornbread mix
- 1 onion
- 1 cup olive oil
- 4 eggs, beaten
- 5 jalapeño peppers
- 1 cup Cheddar cheese
- Salt and pepper, to taste

Chop onions and peppers. Sauté. Mix all ingredients except cheese in a greased casserole dish. Bake at 350° for 35 minutes. Remove from oven and sprinkle grated Cheddar cheese on top.

Ralph N. Brown
First Baptist Church
Lucedale, MS

Meats

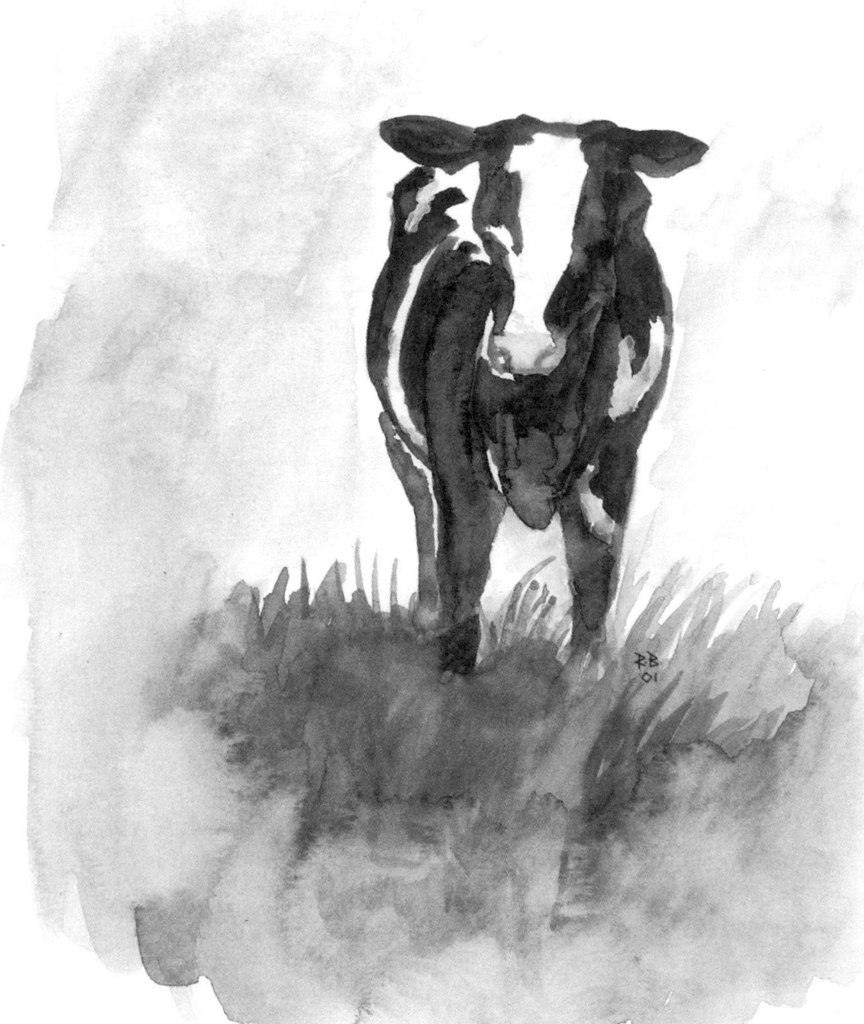

...for tomorrow, and you shall eat meat; Numbers 11:18

MORE

The more you eat the more you want.

- ½ pound noodles
- 1 pound ground beef
- ⅓ cup salad oil
- 1 onion, chopped
- 1 green pepper, chopped
- 1 (10¾-ounce) can tomato soup
- 2 (15½-ounce) cans English peas
- 2 (14¾-ounce) cans cream style corn
- Salt and pepper, to taste
- Grated Cheddar cheese

Cook noodles; drain and rinse. Cook meat in oil until lightly brown. Skim meat out of pan. Cook onion and pepper in oil until soft. Combine meat and noodles. Add tomato soup, peas and corn. Bake in 9 x 13 inch pan for 30 minutes at 350°. May sprinkle grated cheese over top 5 or 10 minutes before removing from oven. Freezes well

Freddy Fisher
Parkway Baptist Church
Kosciusko, MS

ONE POT DINNER

- ¾ pound bacon
- 1 pound ground beef
- 2 (15-ounce) cans pork and beans
- 1 (15½-ounce) can kidney beans
- 1 (15-ounce) can pinto or lima beans
- 1 cup catsup
- ¼ cup brown sugar
- 2 tablespoons liquid smoke or Worcestershire sauce
- 3 tablespoons white vinegar
- ¾ cup chopped onion

Brown ground beef and onions together and drain. Brown bacon. Put all ingredients in crockpot and cook for 4 to 9 hours on low.

Frances Tate
Parkwood Baptist Church
Concord, NC

ROAST BEEF

- 4-5 pounds roast
- ½ stick margarine
- Salt and pepper, to taste
- 6 medium potatoes
- 2 (8-ounce) bottles Catalina French dressing
- 6 carrots
- 1 large onion

Brown roast in margarine in Dutch oven; salt and pepper to taste. Pour dressing over roast. Cover and cook over low heat about 1 hour. Place vegetables around meat. Add enough water to cover vegetables. Cook until vegetables are done.

Erma Morgan
Westlawn Baptist Church
Huntsville, AL

BEEF ROAST

- 2 pounds chuck roast
- 1 (10¾-ounce) can cream of mushroom soup
- 2 cans water
- 1 (1¼-ounce) envelope dry onion soup mix

Mix onion soup and mushroom soup together with 2 cans water. Pour over roast. Cover and bake at 400° for 1 hour.

Dorothy Johnson
First Baptist Church
Avon Park, FL

MANICOTTI

½ pound ground beef
1 clove garlic, crushed
1 cup creamed cottage cheese
4 ounces shredded mozzarella cheese
½ teaspoon salt
½ cup mayonnaise
8 manicotti noodles, cooked and drained
1 (16-ounce) can spaghetti sauce
½ teaspoon oregano
Parmesan cheese

Brown beef and garlic; drain fat. Mix next 4 ingredients in bowl; stir in beef. Fill each manicotti with about ¼ cup cheese-meat filling. Place in 9 x 13 inch baking dish; cover with sauce. Sprinkle with oregano and cheese. Cover with foil. Bake in 350° oven 15 minutes. Remove foil; bake 10 minutes longer or until hot and bubbly.

4 servings

Martha Thetford
Pleasant Garden Baptist Church
Pleasant Garden, NC

GERMAN MEATBALLS

MEATBALLS

2 pounds ground beef
1 cup cracker crumbs
1 (1¼-ounce) envelope dry onion soup mix
3 eggs

Mix ground beef, cracker crumbs, soup mix and eggs together. Make into balls about size of a walnut. Put into 9 x 13 inch baking dish.

SAUCE

1 bottle chili sauce
1 bottle water (use chili sauce bottle)
1 cup brown sugar
1 (14½-ounce) can sauerkraut
1 can whole cranberry sauce

Heat chili sauce, water, sauerkraut and cranberry sauce in saucepan until warm. Pour over meatballs. Bake 2 hours in 350° oven.

Verlon Honeycutt
First Baptist Church
Booneville, MS

BBQ MINI MEAT LOAVES

1 egg
1½ pounds ground turkey, beef or pork
1⅓ cups hickory smoked barbecue sauce
½ cup packaged dry bread crumbs (see note)
⅓ cup chopped fresh flat-leaf parsley
2 tablespoons grated onion
1 clove garlic, finely chopped
½ teaspoon salt

Heat oven to 350°. Beat egg in bowl, mix in beef, ⅔ cup barbecue sauce, crumbs, parsley, onion, garlic and salt. Shape scant ¾ cup mixture into 4 x 2 x 1 inch loaf, for total of 6 loaves. Place on jelly-roll pan or cookie sheet. Top each loaf with about 3 tablespoons of remaining barbecue sauce. Bake in 350° oven for 30 minutes, or until internal temperature registers 160°. Let stand on pan for 10 minutes. Serve immediately or cool completely; refrigerate and serve cold.

For softer-textured meat loaf, substitute 1½ cups soft bread crumbs (2 to 2½ slices white bread).

Evelyn Cox
Skyline Heights Baptist Church
Johnson City, TN

TEX-MEX MEATLOAF

1½ pounds ground beef
3 slices bread, torn into pieces
1 egg
1 (10-ounce) can Rotel
1 small onion chopped
2 teaspoons chili powder
⅓ cup chili sauce

Combine ground beef and next 5 ingredients. Spread into an ungreased 9 x 5 x 2 inch loaf pan. Bake at 375° for 1 hour. Drain excess drippings. Spoon chili sauce over cooked loaf; bake 15 minutes more.

8 servings

Hollie Cartledge
Lincolnton Baptist Church
Lincolnton, GA

SWEET AND SOUR MEAT LOAF

- 1 pound ground chuck
- Salt and pepper, to taste
- 1 cup applesauce
- 1 slice bread, crumbled
- Flour
- ½ cup catsup
- ⅓ cup sugar
- ⅓ cup water

Mix ground chuck, applesauce and bread well and season to taste. Make meatballs the size you want and roll in flour. Bake in 350° oven for about 35 minutes. Remove from oven. Make sauce of catsup, sugar and water and pour over meatballs and bake 30 minutes at 300° until sauce thickens.

Alice Wells
Owensboro, KY

MEAT LOAF

- 1 pound ground beef
- 2 eggs
- ¼ cup catsup
- 1 stack saltines, crushed
- 1 small onion, chopped
- Salt and pepper
- Milk

Mix all ingredients using enough milk to mix everything together well. Put in loaf pan and bake at 300° for 1 hour.

Susan B. Fowler
Clear Spring Baptist Church
Simpsonville, SC

HAMBURGER TATER

1 pound ground beef
1 (1¼-ounce) envelope dry onion soup mix
1 (8½-ounce) can English peas
1 (
1 pa

Spray square pan with Pam. Crumble uncooked ground beef on bottom of square pan. Sprinkle with dry onion soup. Add well drained peas. Then spread with celery soup. Place Tater Tots on top and bake at 350° for 1 hour.

Jane Williamson
First Baptist Church
Estill Springs, TN

COWBELL

1 pound ground beef
2 tablespoons shortening
1 medium onion, chopped
2 (14½-ounce) cans stewed tomatoes
1 tablespoon catsup
1 tablespoon steak sauce
¼ cup chopped green pepper
2 tablespoons chopped parsley (dried)
1 (12 ounce) package elbow macaroni
Salt and pepper, to taste
1 (10¾-ounce) can cream of mushroom soup
1 cup grated cheese

Brown beef in shortening until red color disappears. Add onion, tomatoes, catsup, steak sauce, green pepper and parsley. Simmer for 30 minutes. Cook macaroni according to package directions. Combine macaroni and ground beef mixture in a 9 x 13 inch baking dish. Season to taste. Gently spoon cream of mushroom soup into mixture, lifting from the bottom. Sprinkle grated cheese over top. Bake at 350° for 30 minutes until bubbly and brown

For complete meal, serve with garlic bread and tossed green salad.

Myrtle Campbell
Calvary Baptist Church
Dothan, AL

SY BISQUICK CHEESEBURGER PIE

- pound lean ground beef
- cup chopped onion
- ½ teaspoon salt
- 2 eggs
- ½ cup Bisquick mix
- 1 cup milk
- 1 cup Cheddar cheese, shredded

Grease a 9 inch pie plate. Cook beef and onion together until beef is browned; drain. Spread meat into bottom of pie plate; sprinkle with salt and cheese. Stir remaining ingredients together until well blended. Pour over meat mixture. Bake 25 minutes in 400° oven.

Jeanette Statom
Westlawn Baptist Church
Huntsville, AL

CABBAGE HAMBURGER BAKE

- 1 head cabbage
- 2 pounds hamburger meat
- 1 cup Cheddar cheese, grated
- 2 (10¾-ounce) cans cream of mushroom soup
- Bread crumbs
- 2 tablespoons butter

Slice cabbage and steam until wilted. Spoon into greased casserole dish. Brown hamburger meat lightly. Drain and pour over wilted cabbage. Pour cream of mushroom soup over hamburger. Sprinkle Cheddar cheese over mixture. Melt 2 tablespoons butter and stir in bread crumbs. Crumble over cheese. Bake at 350° for 30 minutes.

Inez Goins
Inwood Baptist Church
Raleigh, NC

CHILI-CORNBREAD PIE

1 pound ground beef
1 large onion, chopped
½ cup bell pepper, chopped
1 tablespoon chili powder
¾ teaspoon black pepper
1 (10¾-ounce) can tomato soup
2 cups water
1 teaspoon salt
1 cup whole kernel corn
½ cup lima beans

CORNBREAD TOPPING
¾ cup cornmeal
1 tablespoon flour
1 tablespoon sugar
½ teaspoon salt
1 egg
½ cup milk
1 tablespoon oil or melted butter

Brown ground beef and drain. Add remaining pie ingredients and simmer, covered, for 20 minutes. Pour into greased 9 x 13 inch bowl and cover with cornbread topping which has been mixed well. Bake at 350° for 20 minutes.

Serve hot with salad or coleslaw for a complete meal.

Eleanor Redd
Chapel Hill Baptist Church
Northport, AL

STROGANOFF

1 pound ground beef
1 onion, chopped
1 (10¾-ounce) can mushroom soup
1 (8-ounce) sour cream
1 (16-ounce) package wide egg noodles

Cook noodles until done. Brown beef and onion and drain. Add mushroom soup and cook until bubbly. Just before serving, add sour cream. Mix with noodles.

Daphne Baldes
New Hope Baptist
Berry, AL

HAMBURGER CHEESE PIE

½ pound ground beef
¼ cup finely chopped onion
1 (9-inch) unbaked pie shell
½ cup grated cheese
2 eggs, well beaten
⅓ cup milk
2 teaspoons cornstarch
¼ teaspoon salt
Pepper
¼ cup mayonnaise

Cook meat and onion until brown. Put on pie shell, then arrange cheese on top. Mix remaining ingredients and spread on top of cheese. Bake in 350° oven for 35 minutes.

Betty Mason
Pine Forest Congregational Christian Church
Valley, AL

HAMBURGER FRY PAN SUPPER

1 pound ground beef
1 medium onion, chopped
2 medium unpeeled red potatoes
2 cups shredded cabbage
2 cups thinly sliced celery
½ cup water
Salt and pepper, to taste

In a large skillet, brown beef and onion; drain. Add remaining ingredients. Cover and simmer for 20 minutes or until vegetables are tender, stirring occasionally.

6 servings

Margaret Carroll
Alabaster, AL

BARBEQUE CUPS

1 pound ground beef
1 tablespoon onion, grated
1 cup grated cheese
½ cup barbeque sauce
1 tablespoon brown sugar
1 package refrigerated biscuits

Brown beef and onions and drain. Add barbeque sauce and sugar. Press biscuits into muffin cups and spoon mixture into cups. Top with grated cheese. Bake in 400° oven for 10 to 12 minutes.

Dean Smith
Derma Baptist Church
Calhoun City, MS

OVEN PORCUPINES

MEATBALLS
1 pound hamburger meat
½ cup regular rice, uncooked
½ cup water
⅓ cup chopped onions
1 teaspoon salt
½ teaspoon celery salt
⅛ teaspoon garlic salt
½ teaspoon pepper

Mix these ingredients well. Make into balls and place in ungreased dish.

SAUCE
1 (15-ounce) can tomato sauce
1 cup water
2 teaspoons Worcestershire sauce

Mix and pour over meatballs and cook 45 minutes in 350° oven covered with foil. Uncover and cook 15 minutes longer.

Estelle [illegible]
Locust Hill Bapt[illegible]
Trave[illegible]

TEXAS HASH

1 small onion
1 pound ground beef
1 teaspoon salt
¼ teaspoon black pepper
1 tablespoon chili powder
1 (14½-ounce) can stewed tomatoes
½ cup Minute rice
Bell pepper (if desired)
½ cup catsup (if needed)

Brown onion in skillet; remove and brown beef. Mix all ingredients together and cut up or mash tomatoes. Pour in 9 x 13 inch pan and bake at 375° for 1 hour covered. Remove top for last 10 minutes. If mixture is too dry, add ½ cup catsup.

Carolyn McIntyre
First Baptist Church
Loretto, TN

LASAGNA

1 pound ground beef
1 medium onion, chopped
1 (14-ounce) Ragu spaghetti sauce with meat
1 (14½-ounce) can diced tomatoes
Garlic, to taste
1 (12-ounce) package lasagna noodles, cooked
1 (3-cup) package mozzarella cheese
1 (16-ounce) carton cottage cheese
1 pound processed cheese loaf, shredded

Brown be[illegible] together. Drain and add next 3 ingredients. Layer [illegible]ese until your 9 x 13 baking inch dish is as full [illegible] cheese layer. Bake at 350° until bubbly.

Ginny Brooks
Parkwood Baptist Church
Concord, NC

STEAK 'N GRAVY

Batter cube steak in flour and brown. Place in
dish. Slice onion and place on top of steak. Mak
browning skillet using water only and pour over s
at 350° for 1 hour or until tender.

Carol Hicks
Mountain View Baptist Church
Bowdon, GA

STEAK AND GRAVY

1 package round steak
2 (10¾-ounce) cans cream of mushroom soup
1 cup water

Cut steak in pieces and place in glass dish. Mix soup and water together and pour over steak. Bake in 350° oven for 1 hour or until meat is tender.

6 to 8 servings

Mildred Strader
Liberty Baptist Church
Madisonville, KY

SALISBURY STEAKS

1½ cups cornflakes
1 egg
⅓ cup barbecue sauce
½ teaspoon salt
⅛ teaspoon pepper
1 pound ground beef
1 medium onion, chopped (optional)

Crush cornflakes; add egg , ¼ cup barbecue sauce, salt and pepper. Mix thoroughly with ground beef. Shape into 6 patties. Place in greased pan, brush with remaining sauce. Bake at 375° for 20 minutes. Do not turn patties while baking.

Jean Hood
Santa Fe Baptist Church
Santa Fe, TN

CUBE STEAK WITH GRAVY

4-6 cube steaks
1 cup flour (set aside 2 tablespoons)
Butter
2 cups water
½ cup milk
Salt and pepper, to taste

Dip cube steaks in flour, shaking off surplus. Place in sizzling hot skillet in which just enough butter to keep meat from sticking has been melted. Pan fry on each side until brown, 4 to 6 minutes. Turn heat down to simmer. Add 1 cup water and let steaks steam for a few minutes. Remove steaks from pan. In pan add mixture of 1 cup cold water, dash salt and pepper, 2 tablespoons flour. (Mix this together before adding to pan). Stir constantly. Add ½ cup milk. Let come to boil. Pour gravy over steaks.

Ginny Brooke
Parkwood Baptist Church
Concord NC

OVEN FRIED CHICKEN

1 fryer-size chicken, cut up
1 stick butter or margarine
1 cup flour
Paprika
Salt and pepper, to taste

Melt margarine or butter in 9 x 13 inch pan. Put cut up chicken in a bag with flour, salt, pepper and paprika. Shake well until chicken pieces are well coated. Put in pan with melted butter; bake at 350° for 45 minutes. Turn over and cook another 30 minutes or until crispy.

This is a great way to cook chicken livers. Cooks in less time.

Ellen Bizzell
St. George Baptist Church
Orangeburg, SC

CRANBERRY CHICKEN

8 boneless chicken breasts
1 (14-ounce) can whole berry cranberry sauce
1 (1¼-ounce) package dry onion soup mix
1 (16-ounce) Catalina dressing

Mix and dry chicken and place in 9 x 13 inch dish. Mix all ingredients together and pour over chicken. Cover dish and refrigerate overnight. Bake at 350° for one hour. Uncover the last 15 minutes.

Makes a wonderful gravy. Serve over rice.

Inez McWhorter
Lincolnton, GA

JOE'S SPICY CHIC N' CROCK

2 chickens, cut in half
2 (1¼-ounce) packages dry onion soup mix
2 tablespoons Cajun Creole seasoning
1 tablespoon all-seasoning salt
1 (10½-ounce) can chicken broth
Salt and pepper, to taste

Pour can of chicken broth in crockpot. Mix salt and pepper and other seasonings in bowl. Rub into chicken with hands. Place chicken in crockpot, sprinkling excess seasoning on top. Cover pot and cook 9- to 10 hours on "low" or until chicken falls apart.

P. Joe Whitt
Reform, AL

CHICKEN PIE

1 whole chicken
1 (10¾-ounce) can cream of chicken soup
1½ (10½-ounce) cans chicken broth
1 cup plain flour
1 teaspoon baking powder
1 stick margarine
1 cup milk

Cook and debone chicken and place into 9 x 13 inch baking dish. Salt and pepper to taste. Heat cream of chicken soup, then add chicken broth and stir until smooth. Pour over chicken. Melt margarine and mix with milk, then add sifted flour and baking powder. Stir until smooth and spoon over chicken mixture. Bake 425° for 30 to 40 minutes or until brown.

Estelle Barnett
Locust Hill Baptist Church
Travelers Rest. SC

CHICKEN TENDERS

- ¾ cup crushed cornflakes
- ¾ cup Parmesan cheese
- 1 (1¼-ounce) envelope ranch dressing mix
- 2 pounds chicken tenders
- ½ cup butter, melted

Put crushed cornflakes, Parmesan and ranch seasoning mix in a zip-top plastic bag with chicken and shake until tenders are coated. Place on lightly greased baking sheet. Bake at 350° for 25 to 30 minutes.

J. Glover
First Baptist Church
Ozark, MO

CHICKEN AND ZUCCHINI SKILLET DINNER

- 1 (14½-ounce) can zucchini
- 1 (10-ounce) can chunk chicken
- 1 (15½-ounce) can whole kernel corn, drained
- 1 (14½-ounce) can garlic and onion diced tomatoes
- 1 small onion, diced
- Vegetable oil spray
- 1 tablespoon vegetable oil

Spray skillet with vegetable spray. Sauté onion in oil. Add zucchini, chicken, corn, diced tomatoes, salt and pepper, to taste. Cook until hot.

Serve with Lettuce and Tomato salad and cornbread

Betty Wilkinson
First Baptist Church
Premont, TX

SOUTHWESTERN CHICKEN

- Boneless chicken breasts, cut into 3-inch strips
- 1 slice bacon for each chicken strip
- ½ teaspoon oregano
- ¼ teaspoon pepper
- ¼ teaspoon garlic powder
- Dill weed, to taste
- 3 cups Kraft 4-grated blend cheese

Mix seasonings together in plastic zip-top bag. Place chicken strips in bag and season well. Remove from bag and wrap a strip of bacon around each strip. Secure with toothpick. Bake at 350° for 30 to 40 minutes. Remove and sprinkle generously with cheese. Return to oven until cheese melts—approximately 5 to 10 minutes.

Annette Thompson
Calvary Baptist Church
Dothan, AL

CARIBBEAN CHICKEN

- 2 large bell peppers
- 4 medium onions
- 3 (20-ounce) cans diced tomatoes
- 2 (14½-ounce) cans pineapple tidbits
- 1 cup flour
- ½ cup sugar
- ½ cup water
- 16 pieces chicken—legs, thighs, wings and breast
- ½ cup vegetable oil
- Salt and pepper, to taste

Slice peppers and onions into strips and sauté in oil. Remove from oil and set aside. Salt and pepper pieces of chicken and brown on both sides in same oil. Remove from oil and set aside Add flour and water, stirring until medium brown. Add diced tomatoes, pineapple and sugar. Pour this mixture into two 9 x 13 inch casserole dishes. Place chicken on top of mixture, then spread peppers and onions evenly. Cover with foil and bake for 1 hour at 350°.

Myrtle S. Potter
Pensacola, FL

MEXICAN CHICK

4-5 chicken breasts
1 large red onion
1 (10-ounce) can tomatoes and green chiles
1 (1
1 (
cheese loa
1 (5½-ounce) bag Dori

Cook and cut chicken into small bite size pieces. Layer in 9 x 13 inch pan, top with red onion rings and processed cheese loaf. Mix tomatoes and soup and pour over layers. Top with crushed Doritos. Bake at 350° until hot and bubbly.

Gail Manly
Northport, AL

CHICKEN QUESADILLAS

1 pound boneless chicken breasts, cubed
1 (10¾-ounce) can Cheddar cheese soup
½ cup chunky salsa
10 (8-inch) flour tortillas

Preheat oven to 425°. Cook chicken in nonstick skillet until well cooked and juices evaporate, stirring often. Add soup and salsa and heat through. Spread about ⅓ cup soup mixture on half of each tortilla to within ½ inch of edge. Moisten edge with water. Fold over and seal. Place on two baking sheets. Bake 5 minutes or until hot.

Serve with Fiesta or Spanish Rice

4 servings

Jeanette Statom
Westlawn Baptist Church
Huntsville, AL

CHICKEN ENCHILADAS

- (10¾-ounce) can cream of chicken soup
- 1 (16-ounce) carton sour cream
- 12 flour tortillas
- 4 chicken breasts
- 1 cup Cheddar cheese
- 1 cup Monterey Jack cheese

Cook, debone chicken and chop. Mix soup and sour cream with small amount of salsa. Place tortillas in microwave to soften (35 to 40 seconds). Spread chicken mixture into center of each tortilla. Add small amount of cheeses on top. Roll up and put in 350° oven. Top with soup mixture and cover with more cheese. Bake until bubbly.

Dorothy Houser
First Baptist Church
Lancaster, TX

CHICKEN AND DUMPLINGS

- 2 cups plain flour
- ½ cup shortening
- 2 eggs
- ½ cup cold water
- ¼ teaspoon salt
- ½ chicken
- 1 (10¾-ounce) can cream of chicken soup
- 4 boiled eggs (optional)

Simmer chicken in enough water to cover until tender. Cool and debone. Add soup to broth. Stir well. In separate bowl, cut shortening into flour. Add eggs (beaten) and cold water to make a stiff dough. Roll out thin and cut into strips. Drop into boiling broth mixture, reduce heat and simmer 15 minutes. Add deboned chicken. Garnish with egg slices if desired.

In loving memory of Imogene Adams

Trillie Brown
Chapel Hill Baptist Church
Northport, AL

CHICKEN PARMESAN

4 skinned, boned chicken breast halves
1/3 cup fine dry bread crumbs
1/2 teaspoon Italian seasoning
1/4 teaspoon dried whole basil
1/8 teaspoon garlic powder
3 tablespoons frozen egg substitute, thawed
Vegetable cooking spray
1 (8-ounce) can tomato sauce
1/4 teaspoon garlic powder
1/4 teaspoon dried whole basil
1/4 cup Parmesan cheese
1/4 cup shredded part-skim mozzarella cheese

Place chicken between 2 sheets of plastic wrap; flatten to 1/4 inch thickness with meat mallet. Combine bread crumbs and next 3 ingredients. Dip chicken in egg substitute; dredge in bread crumb mixture. Coat a large nonstick skillet with cooking spray; place over medium heat until hot. Add chicken and cook 2 minutes or until lightly browned on each side. Place chicken in a 11 x 7 x 2 inch baking dish. Combine tomato sauce, garlic and basil; pour over chicken. Sprinkle with Parmesan cheese. Cover and bake at 350° for 30 minutes. Sprinkle with mozzarella cheese. Bake, uncovered, an additional 5 minutes or until cheese melts.

Norma Burgess
Skyline Heights Baptist Church
Johnson City, TN

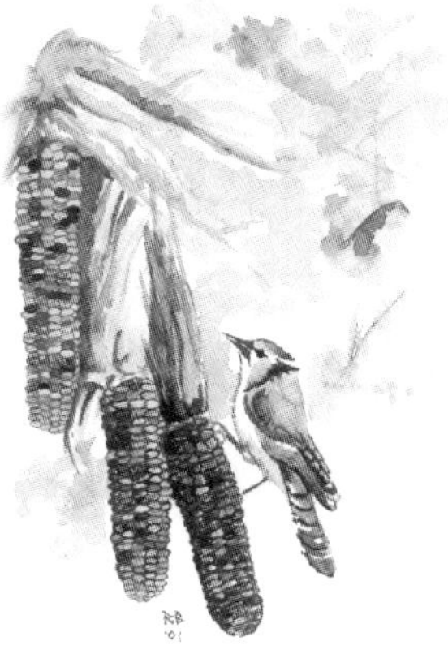

HOT DOG SCRAMBLE

- 1 package wieners, cut in bite-size
- 1 (14½-ounce) can sauerkraut
- 1 (15-ounce) bottle catsup
- 1 (10¾-ounce) can tomato soup
- 1 (14½-ounce) can baked beans
- 1 (16-ounce) can chili without beans
- 1 pound ground beef

Brown beef and drain. Put in crock pot. Add all other ingredients and stir to mix. Cook for about 4 hours.

Drucie Bundrick
First Baptist Church
Troy, AL

RIO GRANDE PORK ROAST

- 1 (3-to 4-pound) boneless pork loin
- ½ cup barbecue sauce
- ½ cup apple or grape jelly
- 1 teaspoon chili powder
- Garlic pepper

Rub surface of roast well with garlic pepper. Place roast in a shallow pan and cook, uncovered, at 350° for 30 minutes. While roast is baking, combine barbecue sauce, jelly and chili powder in small bowl, stirring to mix well. Pour sauce over roast and continue to cook, basting occasionally for 30 more minutes or until meat thermometer registers 155°. Let stand 10 minutes before slicing.

Sue Carter
Flint River Baptist Church
Meridianville, AL

POLISH SAUSAGE DELIGHT

- 1 pound polish sausage
- 10 medium potatoes
- 1 (28-ounce) can sauerkraut
- 1 bay leaf

Cut potatoes in ½-inch rounds and brown. Cover with browned sausage and kraut. Place bay leaf on top. Simmer about 1 hour.

Von Sutton
Lake Catoma Baptist Church
Cullman, AL

THREE ALARM BARBECUE

- 1 2½ pound pork loin roast
- 1 cup cider vinegar
- 1 tablespoon hot sauce
- 1 teaspoon Worcestershire sauce
- 1 teaspoon black pepper
- ¾ teaspoon red pepper
- ½ teaspoon salt

Trim fat from roast. Combine vinegar and remaining ingredients in a large shallow dish or heavy duty zip-loc bag. Add roast; turn to coat. Cover, seal and refrigerate 8 hours, turning occasionally. Remove roast from marinade; set aside, reserving marinade. Prepare smoker to cook. (You may cook in crockpot or in oven.) Pour reserved marinade in a saucepan; cook over medium heat 1 minute to make sauce. Pour over pork; toss well.

Linda Vaughn
Mt. Beulah Baptist Church
Morven, NC

DIFFERENT RIBS

3 pounds pork ribs
3 beef bouillon cubes
1½ cups hot water
⅓ cup honey
5 tablespoons soy sauce
¼ cup sugar
4 teaspoons vinegar
1 teaspoon salt
3 cloves garlic, finely chopped

Cut ribs into serving pieces and place in large zip-loc bag. In a bowl, dissolve bouillon cubes in hot water. Blend in honey, soy sauce, sugar, vinegar, salt and garlic. Pour over ribs. Seal bag and marinate five hours or overnight in refrigerator. Place ribs and marinade in a shallow pan and bake at 350° for 45 minutes or until tender, turning about every 15 minutes.

Sue Carter
Flint River Baptist Church
Toney, AL

SOUTHERN FRIED PIG FEET

Pig Feet

Boil pig feet until done in water with salt and pepper. Soak in vinegar overnight in glass or plastic bowl. Roll in cornmeal and fry until brown and crisp.

Trudy Woodruff
Bowman Baptist Church
Bowman, SC

PORK CHOPS WITH BAKED BEANS

- 1 (16-ounce) can pork and beans
- ½ cup chopped onion
- ¼ cup firmly packed brown sugar
- ¼ cup catsup
- 1 teaspoon prepared mustard
- 4 boneless pork chops
- ¼ cup catsup
- 1 tablespoon brown sugar
- 1 teaspoon Worcestershire sauce

Combine beans and next four ingredients in a lightly greased 2-quart baking dish. Place pork chops on bean mixture. Combine remaining catsup, brown sugar and Worcestershire sauce and spread on chops. Cover and bake 350° for 25 minutes. Uncover and bake 10 minutes.

Lile Dawkins
Mt. Beulah Baptist Church
Wadesboro, NC

SKILLET PORK CHOPS

- 6 pork chops
- 1 cup black coffee
- 1 (10¾-ounce) can cream of mushroom soup
- 1 tablespoon olive oil
- Spices of your choice

Brown pork chops in olive oil. Add coffee and simmer until done. Add cream of mushroom soup and spices. Cover and continue to cook on low for 30 minutes.

Serve over rice if desired.

Rev. Kirby Bunton
First Baptist Church
Windsor, SC

GOURMET PORK CHOPS

2 butterfly pork chops (½- to ¾-inch thick)
1 (10¾-ounce) can cream of celery soup
½ can water
1 can French fried onion rings
Paprika, to taste
Onion salt, to taste
Salt and pepper, to taste
Worcestershire sauce, to taste
Vegetable oil

Season pork chops using Worcestershire sauce, paprika, onion salt, salt and pepper. Brown chops in a small amount of oil. Dilute soup with water. Pour mixture to cover bottom of casserole dish. Place chops in dish and cover with remaining soup. Top with onion rings. Bake at 350° for 1½ hours.

Louis Brown
First Baptist Church
Booneville, MS

PORK CHOP CREOLE

3-4 pork chops
1 (10¾-ounce) can chicken gumbo soup
1 cup flour
Mustard
Salt and pepper, to taste
2 tablespoons vegetable oil

Lay chop on wax paper. Salt and pepper and spread with mustard and flour on one side. Heat oil in a skillet and place chops, mustard and flour side down. After you put in skillet, salt, pepper, mustard and flour the other side of chop (this eliminates a mess preparing). Brown both sides and drain. Add chicken jumbo and enough water to cover chops; simmer for 1 hour or more. This will cook down and will make a thick gravy. Serve on rice.

Marijon Tiller
First Baptist Church
Waverly, TN

PORK CHOPS IN GRAVY

- 1 egg
- 2 tablespoons water
- 8 (½-inch) thick pork chops
- ¾ cup seasoned bread crumbs
- 2 tablespoons vegetable oil
- 1 (10¾-ounce) can condensed cream of mushroom soup
- 1 (10¾-ounce) can condensed French onion soup
- ¼ cup Parmesan cheese

In a shallow bowl, beat eggs and water. Dip pork chops in egg mixture, then coat with bread crumbs. In a large skillet, brown chops in oil. Transfer to a greased 13 x 9 inch baking dish. Combine the soups; pour over chops. Sprinkle with cheese. Cover and bake at 325° for 1½ hours or until meat is tender.

8 servings

Banks Howell
Bay Minette, AL

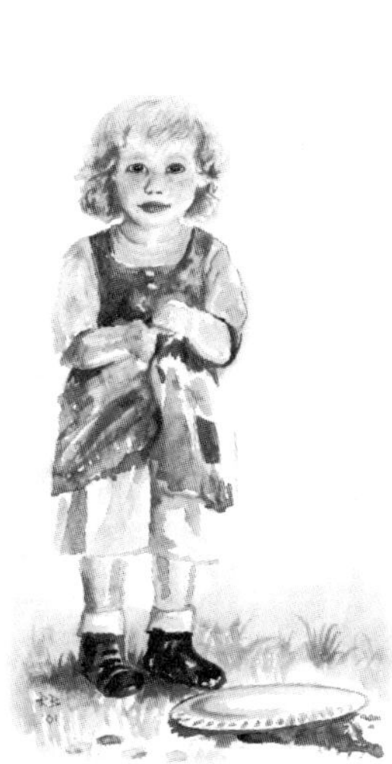

SHRIMP SPAGHETTI

- 2 cups large cooked shrimp
- 2 tablespoons olive oil
- 2 tablespoons margarine
- 3 green onions
- ½ bell pepper
- 1 tablespoon flour
- 4 ounces chicken broth
- 4 ounces half-and-half
- 2 ounces white wine
- Spaghetti noodles to serve 4
- Parmesan cheese

Melt margarine in large skillet and add olive oil. Sauté onions and peppers. While cooking onions and peppers, cook spaghetti noodles and set aside. Add remaining ingredients to onions and pepper. Cook 10 minutes. Drain noodles and add to shrimp mixture. Toss and sprinkle Parmesan cheese over top.

Thin spaghetti is best

Peggy Flippo
First Baptist Church
Slocomb, AL

JAMBALAYA

- 2¼ cups water
- 1½ cups uncooked rice
- 1 (10¾-ounce) can cream of celery soup
- 1 (10¾-ounce) can cream of onion soup
- 1 (10-ounce) can tomatoes and green chiles
- 1 pound smoked sausage
- 1 pound fresh shrimp cleaned

Slice sausage in ½-inch pieces. Combine water, rice, soups, tomatoes and sausage and place in 3-quart shallow baking dish. Cover and bake at 350° for 40 minutes. Stir shrimp into baking dish. Cover and bake 20 minutes.

Serve with French bread—You can omit shrimp and this is still good

Shirley Morgan
Faith Baptist Church
Trinity, AL

CAJUN SHRIMP WITH SPAGHETTI

- 1½ cups butter
- 1 tablespoon lemon juice
- ½ teaspoon basil
- ½ teaspoon thyme
- ¼ teaspoon garlic powder
- 1 tablespoon parsley flakes
- 1 teaspoon salt
- 1 teaspoon pepper
- 1 tablespoon Worcestershire sauce
- 3 pounds cleaned, uncooked shrimp
- 1 (8-ounce) box processed cheese loaf, cut in cubes
- 1 (12-ounce) package spaghetti, cooked

Melt butter in 9 x 13 inch baking dish, add lemon juice and all seasonings. Add shrimp and bake for 25 minutes at 350°, stirring occasionally. Remove from oven and stir in cheese until melted. Stir in spaghetti.

This is better the second day and freezes great

Edna Buff
Calvary Baptist Church
Morganton, NC

SHRIMP ÉTOUFFÉE

- 2 pounds shrimp, peeled and deveined
- ¼ pound margarine or 3 tablespoons oil
- 1 cup chopped onion
- ½ cup chopped celery
- ½ cup chopped bell pepper
- 1 tablespoon cornstarch
- 1½ cups water
- Salt and pepper
- Cayenne pepper

Split shrimp and season with salt, pepper and cayenne pepper to taste. Set aside. Melt margarine or oil and add onion, celery and bell pepper. Cook slowly in an uncovered heavy pot until onions are wilted. Add seasoned shrimp and let simmer, stirring occasionally for 20 minutes. Dissolve cornstarch in water and add to mixture. Cook another 15 minutes, stirring occasionally. Serve over cooked rice.

4 servings

Ethel Freeman
New Chophill Church
West Monroe, LA

SALSA SHRIMP WITH RICE

1 cup long-grain white rice, cooked
½ cup chopped mushrooms, drained
½ cup salsa
1½ ounce shredded Cheddar cheese
1 pound cooked shrimp

Combine all ingredients except cheese. Transfer to microwave safe dish; sprinkle with cheese. Microwave on high 1 minute or until heated through and cheese is melted. Garnish with fresh parsley.

Freddie Anderson
Tabernacle Baptist Church
Macon, GA

LOW COUNTRY SHRIMP BOIL

6 pounds raw shrimp in shells
1 pound butter (save ¾ pound for serving with corn)
½ cup salt
Tabasco sauce, to taste
16 ears corn, broken in half
5 pounds smoked sausage

SAUCE
3 cups catsup
1 teaspoon horseradish
Dash lemon
Dash Worcestershire sauce

Wash and rinse shrimp. Cut sausage into 2- or 3-inch lengths. Fill one 8- to 10-quart pot half full of water. Add ½ cup of butter and salt to water and bring to boil. Add Tabasco sauce, to taste. Put corn in water and boil 5 minutes. Add sausage and boil 2 to 3 minutes. Add shrimp and boil 3 minutes or until shells begin to separate from shrimp. Drain and serve with one large bowl, serving butter with corn and sauce with shrimp.

In the low country, this is often poured on a heap of newspapers, which have been spread on tables. No plates or forks are used, but plenty of paper towels.

Charles Strong, Jr.
Bay Minette, AL

CRAB BREAD

- 2 (6-ounce) cans crab
- 1 (6-ounce) can shrimp
- 1 loaf French bread
- 1 (8-ounce) package cream cheese
- Fresh green onions
- Tabasco sauce
- Tony's Creole seasoning
- Salt and pepper, to taste

Mix drained crab and shrimp with diced green onions and mix all other ingredients. Cut top out of French bread loaf using the subway technique. Fill cavity of bread with mixture and replace top. Wrap in aluminum foil. Bake at 250° for four hours. Can be eaten alone or as a dip with wheat or any other crackers.

Yvonne H. Vining
First Baptist Church
Amite, LA

CRAWFISH ÉTOUFFÉE

- 1 pound crawfish tails
- 2 (10¾-ounce) cans cream of mushroom soup
- ¼ cup butter
- 2 tablespoons Creole seasoning
- 1 cup chopped onions
- 1 cup chopped celery
- 1 cup chopped bell pepper
- ½ cup chopped green onions

Sauté onions, celery and bell peppers in butter until soft. Add crawfish and Creole seasoning. Cook 5 minutes. Add mushroom soup and 2 cups water. Simmer for 10 minutes. Add green onions. Serve over rice.

Paula Barron
Philadelphia Baptist Church
Deville, LA

SALMON LOAF

- 1 (14¾-ounce) can salmon
- ⅓ cup celery, finely chopped
- ⅓ cup onion, finely chopped
- 1 sprig parsley, finely chopped
- ½ cup fine bread crumbs (or more)
- ½ teaspoon celery salt
- ½ cup mayonnaise
- Paprika
- Salt and pepper, to taste

Drain and save liquid from salmon. Combine flaked salmon, bread crumbs, and seasonings with fluid. Mix thoroughly. Pack into small greased loaf pan. Sprinkle generously with paprika. Bake at 350° for 45 minutes.

4 servings

Mrs. Joseph Ryan
Creek Path Baptist
Guntersville, AL

BARBECUED ALASKAN SALMON

- 2 tablespoons butter or margarine
- 2 tablespoons brown sugar
- 1-2 garlic cloves, minced
- 1 tablespoon lemon juice
- 2 teaspoons soy sauce
- ½ teaspoon pepper
- 4 Salmon steaks (1-inch thick)

In a small saucepan, combine all ingredients, except salmon. Cook and stir until sugar is dissolved. Meanwhile, grill salmon, covered, over medium heat for 5 minutes. Turn salmon; baste with the butter sauce. Grill 7 to 9 minutes longer, turning and basting occasionally, or until the salmon flakes easily with a fork.

4 servings

Margaret Carroll
Alabaster, AL

CAJUN SMOTHERED GARFISH BALLS

- 2 pounds fresh garfish
- 1 small bundle of shallots
- 1 white onion
- 1 small bundle of parsley
- 4 slices white bread, soaked in water

Scrape fresh meat off garfish with spoon. Finely chop shallots, onion and parsley and mix with garfish meat and bread. With hands, make small balls (slightly flattened). Roll in flour. Use cast iron pot with lid. Pour in enough oil to fry each ball brown. Remove balls from grease. Pour off excess grease, leaving the brown particles. Add garfish balls back to grease; add ½ cup water. Cover and cook for one hour on medium heat. Do not stir while cooking.

Serve over rice with baked yams.

Bobby Gaspard
Marksville, LA

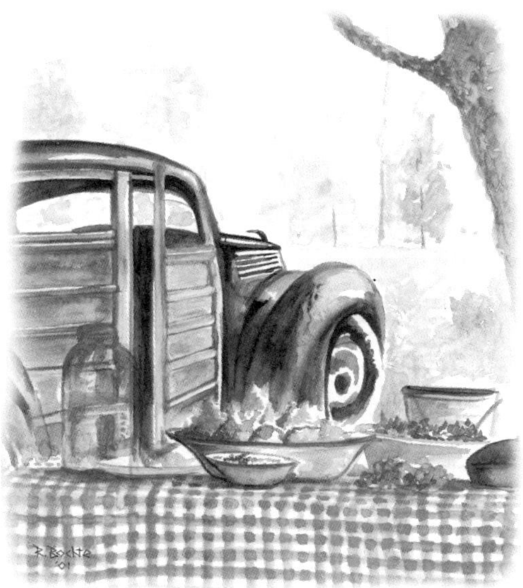

VENISON STEAK

2½ pounds venison (back strap) cut in ½-inch slices
½ cup burgundy cooking wine (optional for gravy)
¾ cup cooking oil
¾ cup flour
1 cup chopped onion
Salt and pepper, to taste
Garlic powder, to taste

Season meat with seasonings. Dredge in flour. Heat oil in heavy frying pan. Brown meat on both sides. Drain well. Reserve 5 tablespoons oil in frying pan. Add 4 tablespoons flour and cook until a golden brown. Add 3 to 4 cups hot water and bring to boil until thickened. Add ½ cup burgundy cooking wine (if desired), meat and onions into the gravy. Cover skillet and cook slowly until tender.

Serve hot with rice or biscuits.

Henry Elmer Peterson
First Baptist Church
Bay Minette, AL

ONION SMOTHERED VENISON

Cut venison in 3-inch pieces. Flour the pieces with garlic, salt, pepper and flour (to individual taste). Fry in small amount of oil on high heat until brown. Drain oil from skillet and cover with water and sliced onions. Cook covered at low heat for approximately 2 hours or until tender.

Linda Dew
First Baptist Church
Pineland, TX

DEER HASH

- 3 pounds cooked and chopped deer meat
- ½ cup brown sugar
- ½ cup vinegar
- 1 teaspoon lemon juice
- 2 medium onions, chopped
- ½ cup catsup
- ½ stick margarine
- 3 tablespoons Worcestershire sauce
- 3 tablespoons mustard
- 2 cups or more broth or water

Mix everything except meat. Cook 20 minutes; add meat and cook slow for 40 minutes. Add enough broth or water to be real moist.

Elizabeth Spruell
Big Creek Church
Williamston, SC

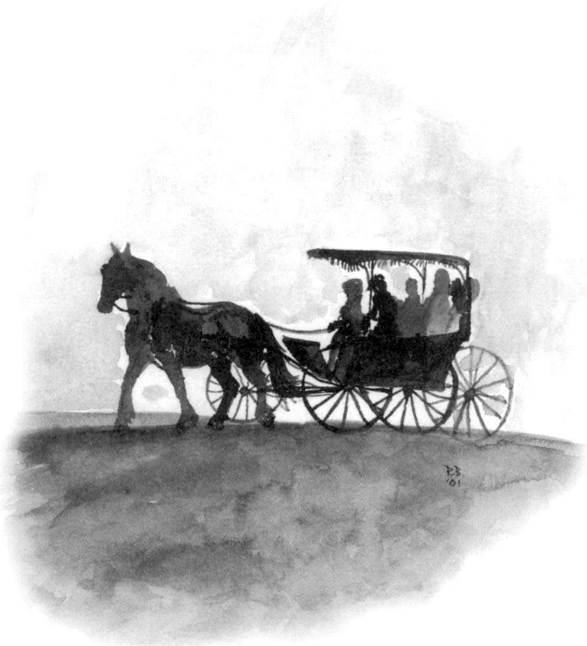

WATER EGGS

2 eggs
½ teaspoon olive oil
Water

Beat eggs and place in pan filled 1-inch deep with boiling water and the olive oil. Stir gently and remove when set. Serve as poached or scrambled eggs.

Elsie Kesner
Lincolnton, NC

ARMADILLO EGGS

12 jalapeño peppers
2 eggs, beaten
Monterrey Jack cheese
Cornmeal
Flour
Salt and pepper

Mix cornmeal, flour, salt and pepper. Stuff peppers with cheese, dip in eggs and dry mix. Deep fry until well browned.

Jim Graves
Hebron Baptist Church
Hebron, MS

BAKED EGGS

6 eggs, lightly beaten
1 pound grated jack cheese
1 cup biscuit mix
1 stick butter or margarine, melted
1 (16-ounce) carton cottage cheese
1 cup milk

Mix together and pour into greased 9 x 13 inch pan. Bake at 350° for 40 minutes

6-8 servings

You may top with diced green chilis, chopped onions, crumbled bacon before baking. Any or all are good. Can be refrigerated or frozen.

Grace A. Tarrant
The Chapel at Lake Wateree
Ridgeway, SC

JALAPEÑO EGGS

8 eggs
½ cup plain flour
¾ teaspoon salt
1 teaspoon baking powder
1 pound Monterey Jack cheese, grated
½ cup cottage cheese

Beat eggs 3 minutes. Combine flour, baking powder and salt. Add to eggs. Stir in cheeses. Pour into greased baking dish. Bake at 350° for 30 to 35 minutes. Let cool 10 minutes before serving.

Don't know where the Jalapeño in title comes from.

Norma Bu
Skyline Heights Baptis
Johns

FRENCH TOAST

1 loaf raisin bread
1 egg per person
Cinnamon
½ gallon vanilla ice cream
5-6 small apples for frying
Whipping cream

Melt ½ gallon ice cream, add eggs and cinnamon. Dip bread in mix and place on grill or pan. While cooking the toast, stir fry apples. Serve toast topped with apples and whipped cream.

Dan Rice
Highland Park Baptist Church
Muscle Shoals, AL

BREAKFAST PIZZA

1 pound sausage
1 can crescent rolls
1 cup frozen hash browns (thawed)
1 cup Cheddar cheese
5 eggs, beaten
¼ cup milk
Salt and pepper, to taste
Parmesan cheese

Cook and drain sausage. Press rolls into pizza pan to make crust. Mix sausage, hash browns, cheese, beaten eggs, milk, salt and pepper together and pour onto dough. Bake at 375° for 25 minutes, then sprinkle with Parmesan cheese and bake 5 minutes longer.

Dean Smith
Derma Baptist Church
Calhoun City, MS

SAUSAGE PIE

- 1 pound sausage, browned
- 1 cup grated Cheddar cheese
- 1 cup milk or half-and-half
- 2 eggs
- 2 (9-inch) pie shells

Combine all ingredients. Pour into pie shells. Bake at 350° for 45 minutes.

Patty Woodham
New Hope Baptist
Fayette, AL

BREAKFAST CASSEROLE

- 1 pound mild sausage
- 6 eggs
- 2 cups milk
- 1 teaspoon dried mustard
- 1 teaspoon salt
- 2 cups cubed bread crusts
- 8 ounces shredded Cheddar cheese

Brown sausage; drain well. Beat eggs; add milk, mustard powder and salt. Blend well; stir in bread crusts, sausage and cheese and mix well. Pour into shallow baking dish. Refrigerate over night. Bake 350° for 45 minutes.

Grace Tarrant
The Chapel at Lake Wateree
Ridgeway, SC

BREAKFAST BAKE

1 can Pillsbury crescent rolls
1 pound sausage, browned and drained
4 eggs, beaten
¾ cup milk
1 cup mozzarella cheese
Salt and pepper

Spread rolls into 9 x 13 inch baking dish to make crust. Add browned sausage Beat eggs with milk, salt and pepper and pour over sausage. Cover with mozzarella cheese. Bake at 350° for 30 minutes.

Gertie Key
Fellowship Baptist Church
Mt. Airy, NC

SAUSAGE AND CHEESE PIE

1 (8-ounce) can crescent rolls
1 pound sausage, browned and drained
2 cups shredded Monterey Jack cheese
4 eggs, slightly beaten
¾ cups milk
2 tablespoons chopped green pepper
½ teaspoon salt
¼ teaspoon pepper
¼ teaspoon oregano

Preheat oven to 400°. Separate crescent dough into 2 large rectangles. Place in ungreased deep dish pie baker, press over bottom and ½ inch up sides to form crust. Seal perforations. Spread scrambled sausage over crust, sprinkle with cheese. Combine remaining ingredients. Pour over cheese. Bake 20 to 25 minutes until golden brown.

6 servings

Dolores Garris
Mt. Beulah Baptist Church
Wadesboro, NC

OVEN DENVER OMELET

- 8 eggs
- ½ cup half-and-half cream
- 1 cup shredded Cheddar cheese
- 1 cup finely chopped, fully cooked mild or hot sausage
- ¼ cup finely chopped green pepper
- ¼ cup finely chopped onion

In a bowl, beat the eggs and cream until light and fluffy. Stir in the cheese, sausage, green pepper and onion. Pour into a greased 9-inch square baking dish. Bake at 400° for 25 minutes or until golden brown.

If you use ham instead of sausage, cook the water out of the ham and pour it off before adding it to the egg mixture. If you do not the water in the ham will cook out during baking and the center of the omelet will not cook because of the water.

4-6 servings

Catherine Carter
Westwood Baptist Church
Alabaster, AL

MACARONI PIE

- 1 cup uncooked macaroni
- 3 eggs, beaten
- 3 cups milk
- ¾ pound (or more) sharp Cheddar cheese
- 2 tablespoons margarine
- Salt and pepper, to taste

Cook macaroni according to directions. Combine eggs and milk in a large bowl, stir in macaroni, cheese and seasoning. Spoon mixture into a 2-quart casserole dish and dot with butter. Bake at 325° for 50 to 60 minutes or until set.

Bonnie B Flemming
Clear Spring Church
Simpsonville, SC

CROCKPOT MACARONI AND CHEESE

- 8 ounce box macaroni, cooked
- 1 stick margarine
- 2 eggs, beaten
- 1 (12-ounce) can evaporated milk
- 1½ cups whole milk
- 3 cups grated cheese
- Salt and pepper, to taste

Turn crockpot on low and let margarine begin to melt. Add cooked macaroni, milk, eggs and 2½ cups grated cheese. Sprinkle ½ cup grated cheese over top. Sprinkle with paprika (optional). Cook on low for 3 hours.

Betty J. Kauffman
Pinewood Baptist Church
Pinewood, SC

CROCKPOT MACARONI AND CHEESE

- 1 (8-ounce) package macaroni, cooked and drained
- 1 (12-ounce) can condensed milk
- 1½ cups regular milk
- 4 cups grated sharp cheese
- 1 stick butter or margarine
- 2 eggs, beaten
- Salt and pepper, to taste

Mix all ingredients except cheese in crockpot. Top with cheese. Cook in crockpot 3 or 4 hours on low temperature.

Ethel Styles
Locust Hill Baptist Church
Travelers Rest, SC

MACARONI AND CHEESE

- 8 ounces small elbow macaroni
- 1 cup sour cream
- 2 cups small curd cottage cheese
- ¼-½ cup buttermilk
- 2 cups grated cheese (medium or sharp Cheddar)
- 1 egg, beaten
- 1 teaspoon salt
- Pepper, to taste

Cook, drain and rinse macaroni. Mix other ingredients. Add macaroni to this mixture. Pour into greased 9 x 13 inch baking dish. Bake at 350° for 45 minutes.

Jerri Garner
Heflin AL

MACARONI CHEESE CASSEROLE

- 1 (4-ounce) box macaroni
- Dash salt
- 2½ cups grated processed cheese loaf
- 1½ cups milk
- 2 eggs
- ¼ cup margarine or butter

Cook macaroni per directions. Layer macaroni and cheese in 9 x 13 inch baking dish. Combine milk, eggs and salt. Beat well. Pour egg mixture over macaroni. Dot with margarine. Bake in preheated oven at 350° for 25 to 30 minutes or until set.

Bobby Sue Green
Trinity Baptist
Childersburg, AL

MACARONI AND CHEESE CASSEROLE

- 1 (8-ounce) package elbow macaroni
- 1 (10¾-ounce) can mushroom soup
- 1 (8-ounce) can sliced mushrooms
- 1 cup mayonnaise
- ¼ cup grated onion
- 1 grated clove of garlic
- ⅓ cup pimentos
- 8 ounce grated Cheddar cheese
- 2 tablespoons margarine

Use directions on package for cooking macaroni. Drain and add margarine, then other ingredients. Bake at 350° for about 30 minutes until heated through.

Margaret Boutwell
First Baptist Church
Bay Minette, AL

PARMESAN ONION BAKE

- 6 medium onions, sliced
- 1 cup diced celery
- 8 tablespoons butter or margarine, divided
- ¼ cup all-purpose flour
- 1 teaspoon salt
- ⅛ teaspoon pepper
- 1½ cups milk
- ⅓ cup Parmesan cheese
- ½ cup chopped pecans

In a large skillet, sauté onions and celery in 3 tablespoons butter until tender. Drain and set aside. In a saucepan, melt the remaining butter, stir in flour, salt and pepper until smooth. Gradually stir in milk. Bring to a boil, cook and stir about 2 minutes until thickened. Pour over vegetables and toss to coat. Pour into an ungreased baking dish. Sprinkle with cheese and pecans. Bake at 350° for 20 to 25 minutes or until heated through. (Do not cover while baking).

6-8 servings

Neola Cleveland
First Baptist Church
Booneville, MS

Desserts

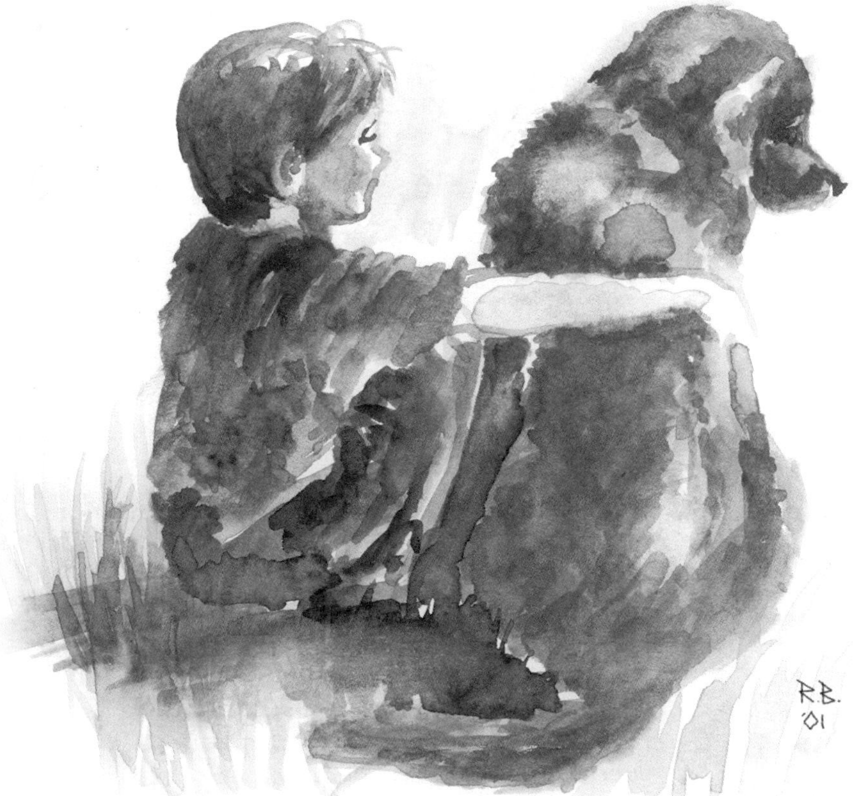

...then I ate it, and it was sweet as honey in my mouth. Ezekiel 3:3

CARAMEL TOPPED OATMEAL CAKE

CAKE

1½ cup boiling water
1 cup quick cooking oatmeal (dry)
1 cup brown sugar, well packed
1 stick margarine
1 cup granulated sugar
2 eggs
1 teaspoon vanilla
1½ cups all-purpose flour
1 teaspoon soda
½ teaspoon salt
1 teaspoon cinnamon

Pour boiling water over oatmeal in bowl. Let stand 20 minutes. Cream margarine, brown sugar and granulated sugar. Add eggs, vanilla and oatmeal mixture. Mix until well blended. Add soda, salt, cinnamon and flour. Pour batter (will be a little thin) into well greased 9 x 13 inch pan. Bake 30 to 40 minutes at 350°.

TOPPING

2 tablespoons butter
1 cup coconut
½ cup brown sugar
⅓ cup evaporated milk, undiluted
½ cup pecans

Combine in saucepan and stir over low heat until well blended. Spread on baked cake and broil until caramelized (brown and crunchy) about 5 minutes.

Frances M. Mabe
Robinhood Road Baptist Church
Winston-Salem, NC

PUMPKIN CHEESE CAKE

2 (8-ounce) packages cream cheese
½ cup pumpkin
½ cup sugar
1 teaspoon vanilla
¼ teaspoon cinnamon
2 eggs
Dash cloves and nutmeg

Mix well and pour into graham cracker crust. Bake 45 minutes at 350°.

Marie Willis
Calvary Baptist Church
Freeport, TX

FRUIT COCKTAIL CAKE

CAKE

- 2 cups plain flour, sifted
- 1 teaspoon soda
- 2 eggs
- 1½ cups sugar
- 1 (30-ounce) can fruit cocktail
- Brown sugar
- Chopped pecans

Combine sugar and eggs, add flour and soda, then add fruit cocktail with juice. Pour into greased and floured pans. Sprinkle the top with brown sugar and chopped pecans. Bake for 30 to 45 minutes at 350° until tests done.

ICING

- ¾ cup sugar
- 1 (3½-ounce) can flaky coconut
- 1 tablespoon flour
- 1 stick margarine
- ½ cup evaporated milk
- 1 teaspoon vanilla

Cream sugar and margarine. Add flour, milk and vanilla. Fold in coconut. Cook 3 or 4 minutes. Do not overcook. Spread while warm.

Martha J. Woodham
Bethel Baptist Church
Dothan, AL

POKE AND POUR CAKE

- 1 (1 pound, 2-ounce) box white cake mix
- 1 (6-ounce) box orange, lime or strawberry Jell-O gelatin
- 1½ cups water
- 1 (12-ounce) carton whipped topping

Bake cake mix according to directions in 9 x 13 inch baking dish. When done, let cool 30 minutes. Mix Jell-O and water and pour over cake that has been poked many times with a fork. Ice with Cool Whip and refrigerate.

12-15 servings

Shirley Cunningham
First Baptist Church,
Estill Springs, TN

RED VELVET CAKE

- 2½ cups cake flour
- 1 teaspoon salt
- 1 teaspoon soda
- 1 (1-ounce) bottle food coloring
- 2 cups sugar
- 1¼ cups Wesson Oil
- 1 cup buttermilk
- 1 teaspoon cocoa
- 1 teaspoon vanilla
- 2 eggs

Sift flour before measuring. Measure and add salt, cocoa and soda. Sift together three times. Mix sugar and oil to blend in large mixing bowl. Add eggs and beat well. Add flour mixture and mix well. Add food color and blend. Add buttermilk and vanilla. Blend well. Pour into 2 well greased and floured 9-inch pans and bake at 350° for 25 to 30 minutes or until cake tests done with toothpick.

Jeanette Hollis
Prattville, AL

EGG-LESS, MILK-LESS, BUTTER-LESS CAKE

- 1 cup brown sugar, firmly packed
- 1¼ cups water
- ½ cup shortening
- 1½ cups raisins
- 2 cups all-purpose flour, sifted
- ½ teaspoon baking soda
- 1 teaspoon baking powder
- ½ teaspoon salt
- 1 teaspoon cinnamon
- 1 teaspoon nutmeg
- 1 cup nuts, chopped
- 1 teaspoon orange or lemon peel, grated

In saucepan, combine brown sugar, water, shortening and raisins; bring to a boil and cook 3 minutes. Cool. Onto a square of waxed paper, sift together flour, baking soda, baking powder, salt and spices. Add nuts and orange or lemon peel. Mix all ingredients together and pour batter into a greased and floured loaf pan. Bake in a 350° heated oven for 45 minutes. Remove cake from pan and place on rack to cool.

Alice Lawrence
Stetson Baptist Church
Deland FL

CHOCOLATE ÉCLAIR CAKE

- 1 cup powdered sugar
- 1 (10-ounce) carton Cool Whip
- 2 (3.4-ounce) boxes vanilla or banana instant pudding mix
- 3 cups milk
- 1 box graham crackers
- 1 can milk chocolate icing

Mix milk and pudding. Add sugar and beat. Fold in Cool Whip. Mix as you would banana pudding. Break graham crackers in half and put a layer on bottom of 9 x 13 inch cake pan. Put about one-half the pudding mixture on the crackers, spreading evenly. Put another layer of crackers, the rest of pudding mixture and top with another layer of crackers. Put the icing into the microwave long enough to soften it. Pour on top of the crackers and spread to cover. Place in the refrigerator overnight.

Patsy Smith
Amite, LA

ONE BOWL CHOCOLATE CAKE

- 2 cups all-purpose flour
- 2 cups sugar
- ½ cup baking cocoa
- 2 teaspoons baking soda
- 1 teaspoon baking powder
- ½ teaspoon salt
- 1 cup vegetable oil
- 1 cup buttermilk
- 2 eggs
- 1 cup hot water
- Frosting of choice

In a large bowl, combine dry ingredients. Stir in oil, buttermilk and eggs. Add water and stir until combined. Pour into greased 9 x 13 inch baking pan. Bake at 350° oven for 35 to 38 minutes or until a toothpick inserted near the center comes out clean. Cool completely. Frost.

Margaret Carroll
Alabaster, AL

CHOCOLATE SHEET CAKE

CAKE

- 2 sticks margarine
- 1 cup water
- 3½ tablespoons cocoa
- ½ cup buttermilk
- 2 eggs
- 2 cups granulated sugar
- 2 cups plain flour
- ½ teaspoon salt
- ½ teaspoon soda

In saucepan, heat margarine, water and cocoa. Sift flour, salt and soda together. In mixer, beat buttermilk, eggs and sugar. Add flour mixture, alternating with melted chocolate to mixer ingredients. Will make thin batter. Bake in 9 x 13 inch pan at 375° approximately 20 to 25 minutes until tests done.

ICING

- 3½ tablespoons cocoa
- ⅓ cup buttermilk
- 1 stick margarine
- 1 box powdered sugar

Heat buttermilk, margarine and cocoa until melted. In mixer, combine this mixture with powdered sugar until smooth. Pour on cake while slightly warm.

Sometimes there is too much icing. I add a little peanut butter and roll into bite size balls to make delicious candy.

France M. Mabe
Robinhood Road Baptist Church
Winston-Salem, NC

DELICIOUS CHOCOLATE CAKE

CAKE

1 (1 pound, 2-ounce) box Swiss chocolate cake mix

Mix according to instructions on box except to bake in 3 cake pans at 350° for 20 minutes.

ICING

½ cup granulated sugar
1 cup powdered sugar
10 Hershey candy bars with almonds, chopped
1 (8-ounce) package cream cheese
1 (12-ounce) carton Cool Whip

Cream cheese and sugars; add chopped candy bars. Fold in Cool Whip. Ice cake and garnish with 2 chopped Hershey bars.

Mary Morrison
Lineville Baptist Church
Lineville, AL

CHOCOLATE MARSHMALLOW CAKE

CAKE

- 1½ cups butter
- 1½ cups sugar
- 1½ cups self-rising flour
- 1½ cups nuts
- 3 tablespoons cocoa
- 3 eggs
- 1 teaspoon vanilla
- 1 package miniature marshmallows

Cream butter and sugar. Add cocoa. Add eggs, one at a time, beating well after each. Add flour, nuts and vanilla. Mix well. Pour batter into a greased and floured 9 x 13 inch baking dish. Bake at 325° for 40 minutes. Remove from oven and spread marshmallows over hot cake. When cool, spread frosting over top.

FROSTING

- 1 stick margarine
- 4 tablespoons cocoa
- 6 tablespoons milk
- 1 (16-ounce) box powdered sugar
- 1 teaspoon vanilla

Combine margarine, cocoa and milk in saucepan and mix. Bring to a rapid boil. Remove from heat and add sugar and vanilla and beat until smooth.

Norma Burgess
Skyline Heights Baptist Church
Johnson City, TN

MYSTERY GERMAN CHOCOLATE CAKE

- 1 (1 pound, 2-ounce) box German Chocolate Cake mix
- 1 cup plain flour
- ½ cup sugar
- 1 teaspoon baking powder
- 5 eggs
- ½ cup cooking oil
- 1 cup water
- 1 bag Bits-of-Brickle
- 1 cup chopped pecans
- 1 stick margarine
- 1 (8-ounce) package cream cheese
- 1 egg
- 1 (16-ounce) box powdered sugar
- 1 teaspoon vanilla

Mix cake mix and next six ingredients and beat two minutes. Line a 10 by 15 inch baking pan and grease and flour well. Sprinkle brickle and pecans over bottom of pan. Pour cake mix over this mixture. Melt margarine and then mix with cream cheese and powdered sugar. Add slightly beaten egg and vanilla. Drizzle sugar mixture on top of cake mix. Bake in 350° heated oven for 45 to 50 minutes. Cake is done when toothpick stuck in middle comes out clean.

Fred Guthrie
Westwood Baptist Church
Alabaster, AL

EVER SO EASY FRUITCAKE

- 2½ cups unsifted flour
- 1 teaspoon baking soda
- 2 eggs, slightly beaten
- 1 (28-ounce) jar None-Such Ready-to-Use Mincemeat
- 1 (14-ounce) can sweetened condensed milk
- 2 cups mixed candied fruit
- 1 cup coarsely chopped pecans

Generously grease and flour two 8.5 x 5 inch loaf pans. Sift together flour and baking soda; set aside. In large bowl, combine remaining ingredients; blend in dry ingredients. Pour into prepared pans. Bake in 300° heated oven for 65 to 70 minutes, or until toothpick inserted near center comes out clean. Cool 15 minutes. Turn out of pan. Cool thoroughly and refrigerate or freeze.

Jeanette Staton
Westlawn Baptist Church
Huntsville, AL

JELL-O CAKE

1 (1 pound, 2-ounce) box white cake mix
¾ cup water
¾ cup oil
1 teaspoon vanilla flavoring
1 teaspoon lemon flavoring
1 (3-ounce) box lemon Jell-O
6 eggs

Mix all ingredients with mixer until well blended. Cook in well greased and floured Bundt pan at 325° for about 30 to 40 minutes until tests done.

Ann Smith
New Hope Baptist Church
Berry, AL

7-UP POUND CAKE

2 sticks margarine
½ cup shortening
3 cups sugar
5 eggs
1 teaspoon lemon extract
1 teaspoon vanilla
3 cups all-purpose flour
1 (7-ounce) bottle 7-Up

Cream butter and shortening with sugar. Add eggs one at a time, beating after each addition. Add lemon and vanilla flavorings. Add flour and 7-Up alternately, beating after each addition. Bake in a greased and floured tube pan at 300° for 1½ hours, or until cake tests done.

Betty J. Kauffman
Pinewood Baptist Church
Pinewood, SC

FIVE FLAVOR POUND CAKE

1 cup butter
½ cup Crisco shortening
3 cups sugar
3 cups plain flour
1 cup milk
1 teaspoon baking powder
5 eggs
1 teaspoon vanilla flavoring
1 teaspoon lemon flavoring
1 teaspoon rum flavoring
1 teaspoon almond flavoring
1 teaspoon coconut flavoring

Cream butter, Crisco and sugar. Add eggs. Sift flour and baking powder. Add alternately with milk; add flavoring and pour into tube pan. Bake at 350° for 1 hour and 20 minutes.

Betty Carpenter
Lincolnton, NC

CHOCOLATE MILK POUND CAKE

1 pound butter
½ cup Crisco
3 cups sugar
6 eggs
3 cups plain flour
½ teaspoon baking powder
1 cup chocolate milk
¼ cup Hershey cocoa
2 teaspoons vanilla flavoring

Soften butter and Crisco add sugar and beat well. Add eggs one at a time. Sift flour and baking powder together. Add flour and cocoa. Mix well. Pour in chocolate milk a little at a time; add vanilla. Place in cold oven and bake at 325° for 1½ hours or until done.

Imogene Fowler
Fairview Street Baptist Church
Fountain Inn, SC

POUND CAKE

2 cups Crisco
2¾ cups sugar
3¾ cups plain flour
9 eggs
1 tablespoon butter flavoring
1 tablespoon vanilla flavoring
7 tablespoons water

Cream sugar and Crisco; add eggs, beating well after each egg. Add flavoring and water; beat, add flour and beat until well blended. Bake in greased tube pan for 1 hour and 20 minutes at 325°.

Opal Ferguson
Enon Baptist Church
Danville, AL

MILLION DOLLAR POUND CAKE

1 pound butter, softened
3 cups sugar
6 eggs
4 cups all-purpose flour
¾ cup milk
1 teaspoon almond extract
1 teaspoons vanilla

Cream butter, gradually adding sugar and beating well. Add eggs one at a time beating after each addition. Add flour, alternating with milk. Mix until well blended. Stir in flavorings. Pour into a greased and floured 10-inch tube pan. Bake at 300° for 1 hour and 40 minutes.

Elizabeth Mendenhall
Deland, FL

HANNAH'S POUND CAKE

- 1 (8-ounce) package cream cheese
- 2½ sticks butter
- 3 cups sugar
- 6 large eggs
- 3 cups all-purpose flour
- 2 pinches baking powder
- 2-3 teaspoons lemon or coconut flavoring

Everything should be at room temperature. Beat cream cheese and butter together for 5 minutes; add sugar and beat 5 more minutes. Add eggs one at a time and beat. Gradually add flour and baking powder and mix. Add flavoring last and mix. Bake in greased and floured tube pan. Start cake in cold oven and bake at 300° for 1 hour and 30 minutes.

Ann Cherry
Mt. Gilead Baptist Church
Dothan, AL

BAPTIST POUND CAKE

- ½ cup shortening
- 1 stick margarine
- 3 cups sugar
- 5 eggs
- 3 cups flour
- ½ teaspoon baking powder
- 1 cup milk
- 1 teaspoon vanilla or lemon extract

Cream shortening and margarine with sugar. Add one egg at a time, beating well with mixer after each addition. Sift flour and baking powder together. Sift again. Add flour and milk alternately. Mix well. Add extract. Pour into greased and floured tube pan. Place in cold oven and bake at 350° for 1 hour and 30 minutes.

Barbara Walker
First Baptist Church
Worthington, KY

BLUEBERRY POUND CAKE

1 cup butter
2¼ cups sugar
4 eggs
1 teaspoon vanilla
3 cups flour
2 teaspoons baking powder
½ teaspoon salt
2 cups blueberries

Grease and flour tube or Bundt pan; sprinkle with sugar. Cream butter, sugar, eggs, vanilla, flour and baking powder. Flour blueberries and fold into mixture. Bake at 325° for 1 hour and 10 minutes. Cool 10 minutes before removing from pan.

Jane Williamson
First Baptist Church
Estill Springs, TN

CHOCOLATE SOUR CREAM POUND CAKE

1½ cups softened butter
3 cups sugar
5 eggs
3 cups plain flour
½ cup cocoa
1 teaspoon baking soda
¼ teaspoon salt
1 (8-ounce) carton sour cream
1 cup boiling water
2 teaspoons vanilla flavoring

Cream butter, gradually add sugar and beat well. Add eggs one at a time, beating well after each one. Combine flour, cocoa, soda and salt; add to cream mixture alternately with sour cream beginning and ending with flour mixture. Add boiling water and vanilla. Bake at 350° for 1 hour. Use Bundt or tube cake pan.

Jan Rimmer
Stony Point, NC

HUNGARIAN SOUR CREAM COFFEE CAKE

- ½ pint sour cream
- 1½ teaspoons baking powder
- 1 teaspoon baking soda
- ¼ pound butter
- 1 cup sugar
- 2 eggs
- 1½ cups sifted all-purpose flour
- ½ cup sugar
- 1 teaspoon cinnamon
- 3 tablespoons chopped nuts

Mix sour cream, baking powder and baking soda together and set aside. Cream butter and sugar until smooth; add eggs and sour cream mixture to batter. Little by little add flour to mixture. Set aside and mix ½ cup sugar, cinnamon and chopped nuts together. Pour half the batter into greased pan, then half the sugar, cinnamon and nut mixture, then rest of batter and rest of nut mixture. Cut through with a knife (like a marble cake). Bake at 325°for 40 to 45 minutes in a greased 8-inch square cake pan.

Moist and good warm or cold

Margaret Bowne
St. Luke United Methodist Church
Pensacola, FL

SAD CAKE

- 1 package biscuit mix
- 4 eggs
- 1 cup pecans
- 1 (16-ounce) box brown sugar
- 1 (3½-ounce) can flaked coconut
- 1 cup Wesson Oil

Put all in mixing bowl and mix well. Pour into greased pan and bake at 350° for 45 minutes. Cool and cut into squares.

Carolyn Strickland
Ridgecrest Baptist Church
Dothan, AL

CREAM SICKLE CHEESE CAKE

- 2 (8-ounce) packages cream cheese
- ½ cup sugar
- 2 eggs
- ¾ cups sour cream
- 1 teaspoon vanilla
- 1 teaspoon orange extract
- 2 drops yellow food coloring
- 1 drop red food coloring
- 1 (9-inch) graham cracker crust

Beat cream cheese and sugar until fluffy. Add eggs; beat well. Add sour cream and vanilla and beat well. Place 1 cup in small bowl and stir in extract and coloring. Pour remaining cream cheese in pie crust. Drop in orange mixture and swirl. Bake 30 to 35 minutes in 350° oven until slightly firm around edges. Center will be slightly loose. Allow to cool 1 hour and then chill several hours.

Can top with dollops of whipped cream and slices of oranges if desired.

Lillie Phillips
Wayside Baptist Church
Miami, FL

DOWN SOUTH YAM CAKE

- 2 cups sugar
- 1 cup margarine (softened)
- 1½ teaspoons vanilla
- 5 eggs
- 1¼ cups mashed, cooked yams
- 2 teaspoons cinnamon
- 2 cups self-rising flour
- ½ teaspoon soda
- ½ teaspoon nutmeg
- 1 cup chopped nuts
- 1 cup raisins
- 1 (8-ounce) can crushed pineapple, drained
- 1 can Pillsbury Coconut and Pecan Frosting

Grease and flour 10-inch tube pan. In large bowl, cream sugar, butter and vanilla until light and fluffy; add eggs one at a time, beating well after each addition. Add yams to creamed mixture, beating until well mixed. Add flour, cinnamon, soda and nutmeg; mix well. By hand, fold in nuts, raisins and pineapple; spoon butter into pan and spread evenly. Place in a warm 325° oven and bake for 60 to 70 minutes or until evenly browned. Cool completely and frost.

Rudy Branham
Sawney's Creek Baptist Church
Elgin, SC

DOROTHY'S GEORGIA PEACHES AND CREAM CAKE

CAKE

- 1 (1 pound, 2-ounce) butter cake mix
- 1 (8-ounce) carton sour cream
- ⅓ cup cooking oil
- ¼ cup sugar
- ¼ cup water
- 4 eggs

Blend ingredients and beat at high speed for 3 minutes. Pour into 2 well greased and floured 9 inch cake pans and bake in 375° oven for 30 minutes or until tests done. Cool completely and split layers to make 4 layers.

FILLING

- 2 cups sour cream
- 2 cups powdered sugar
- 1 (12-ounce) carton whipped topping
- 2-3 cups fresh sliced peaches

Combine and mix sour cream, powdered sugar and whipped topping. Stack cake layers using lots of filling and top each layer with sliced peaches. Cover sides of cake with whipped topping mixture and refrigerate.

Willene Holton
First Baptist Church
Alma, GA

APPLE BRUNCH CAKE

- 2 cups peeled, chopped apples
- 1¼ cups sugar
- 1 egg
- 1½ cups all-purpose flour
- 1 teaspoon baking soda
- ½ teaspoon salt
- ½ teaspoon cinnamon
- ½ teaspoon allspice
- ½ teaspoon nutmeg
- ½ cup raisins
- ½ cup chopped nuts

Pour sugar over chopped apples and let stand 10 minutes. Mix flour, salt and spices. Add egg to apples, then add flour mixture. Add raisins and nuts. Pour into 9 x 13 inch pan and bake at 350° for 20 to 25 minutes.

Evelyn Leatherwood
Fleming Baptist Church
Richmond Hill, GA

MEXICAN FRUIT CAKE

CAKE

2 cups sugar
2 cups self-rising flour
2 eggs
1 (20-ounce) can crushed pineapple, in heavy syrup
½ teaspoon baking soda
1 cup pecans

Mix all together and pour into 9 x 13 inch baking pan and bake for 30 minutes or until brown at 350°.

ICING

1 stick margarine
1 (8-ounce) package cream cheese
2 cups powdered sugar
1 teaspoon vanilla
½ cup pecans

Mix all together and pour mixture over hot cake.

Becky May
Macedonia Baptist Church
Mendenhall, MS

STRAWBERRY PUNCH BOWL CAKE

1 (1 pound, 2-ounce) package strawberry cake mix
1 (20-ounce) can crushed pineapple
2 (3.4-ounce) boxes instant vanilla pudding mix
1 (10-ounce) carton whipped topping
1 cup pecans, chopped

Mix cake mix as directed on box. Bake making 2 layers. Crumble one layer in truffle bowl. Mix pudding as directed on box. Pour ½ over first layer. Repeat with second layer, adding pineapple. Spread Cool Whip on top. Top with chopped pecans.

Nell Lushner
Greenville, SC

SWEDISH PINEAPPLE CAKE

CAKE

- 2 cups sugar
- 1 (20-ounce) can crushed pineapple
- 1 cup chopped pecans
- 1 teaspoon vanilla
- 2 cups self-rising flour
- 1 teaspoon soda

Mix ingredients in order by hand. Pour into ungreased, unfloured 9 x 13 inch pan. Bake at 350° for 30 minutes or until toothpick stuck in middle is clear.

ICING

- 1 (8-ounce) package cream cheese, softened
- 1 stick margarine, melted
- ¾ cup sugar
- 1 cup chopped pecans

Stir sugar into margarine until dissolved; add remaining ingredients and mix well. Spread on cake immediately after removing from oven.

Christine Coleman
Macedonia Baptist Church
Mendenhall, MS

PEAR PRESERVE CAKE

- 1 cup shortening
- 2½ cups sugar
- 4 large eggs
- 1 teaspoon vanilla
- 3¼ cups all-purpose flour
- ¾ teaspoon soda
- 1 teaspoon cinnamon
- 1 teaspoon cloves
- 1 teaspoon allspice
- 1 cup buttermilk
- 1 pint pear preserves
- 1 cup chopped pecans

Mix all ingredients together except for preserves and pecans. When well mixed, fold in preserves and pecans. Pour into tube pan and bake at 325° for 1 hour and 30 minutes.

Mildre
Da

JUDY'S DELIGHTFULLY NUTTY PECAN PIE CAKE

- 1 (1 pound, 2-ounce) yellow cake mix
- 1 stick butter, melted
- 4 medium eggs
- 1½ cups light corn syrup
- ½ cup dark brown sugar, packed
- 1 teaspoon vanilla extract
- 2 cups toasted, chopped pecans

Place cake mix, melted butter and 1 egg in large mixing bowl. Beat on low speed for 30 seconds until well blended. Measure out ⅔ cup of batter; set aside. Spread remaining batter in bottom of ungreased 9 x 13 x 2 inch baking dish. Bake for 15 minutes or until top lightly browns. Remove dish to cooling rack. Place remaining batter, corn syrup, sugar and remaining 3 eggs and vanilla in a large bowl. Beat with mixer on medium speed for 1 minute; stop mixer, scrape bowl down, beat 1 more minute. Fold in the pecans. Pour pecan mixture on top of warm cake. Gently smooth out evenly over cake. Bake in 325° oven for 40 minutes or until the edges are brown but the middle is still soft. Remove to wire rack and cool for 35 minutes. Slice and serve with vanilla ice cream.

Judy David
Northside Baptist Church
Lafayette, LA

BABY FOOD CAKE

- 1 (1 pound, 2-ounce) yellow cake mix
- 4 eggs
- ½ cup sugar
- 2 medium jars baby food (fruit your choice)
- ¾ cups oil

Mix well and pour into Bundt pan and bake 1 hour at 325°.

Lois Sisk
Vale, NC

FRESH APPLE CAKE WITH COCONUT ICING

CAKE

- 2 cups sugar
- ⅔ cups oil
- 3 eggs, beaten separately
- 3 cups self-rising flour
- 1 teaspoon vanilla
- 3 cups chopped apples
- 1 cup chopped pecans
- ¾ cup orange juice

Mix all ingredients together except for orange juice. Place in 3 layer pans and bake in 350° oven for 40 to 45 minutes. Punch holes in layers and pour ¼ cup orange juice over each layer before icing.

ICING

- 1 cup granulated sugar
- 1 cup powdered sugar
- 1 (8-ounce) package cream cheese
- 1 (12-ounce) carton frozen whipped topping
- 1 (5-ounce) package frozen coconut

Mix all ingredients together except for coconut and beat well. Spread over each layer. Sprinkle coconut over each layer after icing.

Avis Hall
Angier Baptist Church
Angier, NC

PINEAPPLE CAKE

CAKE

- 1 (1 pound, 2-ounce) package yellow cake mix
- 4 eggs
- 1 (3.4-ounce) box vanilla or lemon instant pudding mix
- ⅓ cup Wesson Oil
- 1 cup water

Mix and bake in Bundt or tube pan for 1 hour at 350°

ICING

- 1 cup sugar
- 1 (6-ounce) can pineapple juice

Mix and bring to boil on stove (to melt sugar). Stick cake with tooth picks and pour above over cake. Let set until cool and remove from pan.

Barbara Stewart
Westmeade Baptist Church
Decatur, AL

JAM CAKE

3 cups flour
1 teaspoon baking soda
½ teaspoon salt
3 teaspoons allspice
2 teaspoons cloves
3 teaspoons cinnamon
1 stick melted margarine
3 eggs
1 cup buttermilk
2 cups dark Karo syrup
1 cup blackberry jam
1 cup strawberry preserves
1 cup nuts
1 cup seeded raisins, floured

Mix all ingredients together. Bake at 350° for 1 hour or until straw comes out clean. Bake in 3 pans.

Faustine Gritton
Hopewell Baptist Church
Harrodsburg, KY

RAW APPLE CAKE

2 cups sugar
3 cups flour
1½ cups Wesson Oil
3 eggs
1 teaspoon soda
1 teaspoon cinnamon
1 teaspoon salt
1 cup chopped black walnuts
3 cups raw, juicy apples, chopped
1 teaspoon vanilla
1 cup raisins
½ cup coconut

Mix all ingredients. Pour into Bundt pan and bake 1 hour and 30 to 45 minutes on 325°.

Edna Buff
Calvary Baptist Church
Morganton, NC

STRAWBERRY CAKE

CAKE

- 1 (1 pound, 2-ounce) cake mix
- 4 eggs
- ½ cup water
- 3 teaspoons flour
- 1 (3-ounce) box strawberry Jell-O gelatin
- 1 cup vegetable oil
- ¾ cup strawberries, mashed

Mix all ingredients except strawberries. Add them last. Pour into tube pan and bake 60 minutes at 350°.

ICING

- 1 (1 pound) box powdered sugar
- 1 stick margarine
- ¼ cup mashed strawberries

Mix together and pour over cooled cake.

Joanna Sheetz
Parkwood Baptist Church
Concord, NC

BANANA NUT CAKE

- 1½ cups sugar
- 2 cups self-rising flour
- 2 eggs
- 1 cup Wesson Oil
- ½ teaspoon baking soda
- 3 real ripe bananas, mashed
- 1½ cups pecans, chopped fine

Put all ingredients in a bowl and mix by hand until blended. Put in a greased and floured tube pan. Bake at 350° about 45 to 50 minutes until done.

Jo Williams
First Baptist Church
Amite, LA

PISTACHIO CAKE

CAKE

- 1 (1 pound, 2-ounce) box white cake mix (not pudding kind)
- ¾ cup vegetable oil
- 3 eggs
- 1 cup lemon-lime or club soda
- 1 (3.4-ounce) package Pistachio instant pudding mix
- 1 cup chopped pecans
- ½ cup coconut

Combine cake mix and next 4 ingredients, mixing well. Stir in pecans and coconut. Bake in 9 x 13 inch pan at 350° for 45 minutes.

ICING

- 2 envelopes Dream Whip topping
- 1½ cups milk
- 1 (3.4-ounce) package Pistachio instant pudding mix
- ¾ cups chopped pecans
- ½ cup coconut

Combine Dream Whip, milk and pudding mix; beat until thick. Sprinkle with pecans and coconut. Spread on cooled cake.

Juanita Almond
Parkwood Baptist Church
Concord, NC

VANILLA WAFER CAKE

- 1 box vanilla wafers
- 1 (12-ounce) can skimmed or low-fat milk
- 3 cups sugar
- 6 eggs
- 5 ounces frozen coconut
- 1 cup pecans, chopped fine

Mix all ingredients together and bake at 350° for 35 to 45 minutes or until done.

Beth Gower
Bethel Baptist Church
Chesapeake, VA

BLUEBERRY PUDDING CAKE

CAKE

- 2 cups fresh or frozen blueberries
- 1 teaspoon cinnamon
- 1 teaspoon lemon juice
- 1 cup all-purpose flour
- ¾ cup sugar
- 1 teaspoon baking powder
- ½ cup milk
- 3 tablespoons butter, melted

Toss blueberries with cinnamon and lemon juice. Place in a greased 8-inch square baking pan. Combine flour, sugar and baking powder; stir in milk and butter and spoon over berries. Combine sugar and cornstarch and sprinkle over batter. Slowly pour boiling water over all ingredients. Bake at 350° for 45 to 50 minutes or until the cake tests done.

TOPPING

- ¾ cup sugar
- 1 tablespoon cornstarch
- 1 cup boiling water

Thicken and pour over cake when cooled.

Marguerite Nicholson
Russellville, AL

DIRT CAKE

- 1 (8-ounce) cream cheese
- 1 (12-ounce) carton Cool Whip
- 1 cup powdered sugar
- 1 stick margarine

Soften and cream together above ingredients:

- 2 (3.4-ounce) boxes vanilla instant pudding
- 1 (16-ounce) package Oreo cookies

Mix pudding according to package. Then mix with the cream cheese mixture. Crush cookies. Layer in flower pot or dish with crushed cookies on bottom; then creamy mixture and then layer of cookies on top.

Peggy McCord
Bethel Baptist Church
Dothan, AL

ORANGE SURPRISE CAKE

CAKE

- 1 (1 pound, 2-ounce) box yellow cake mix
- 1 (11-ounce) can mandarin oranges
- 4 eggs
- ½ cup vegetable oil

Mix together and bake at 350° for 35 minutes or until done. Cool.

FROSTING

- 1 (20-ounce) can crushed pineapple
- 1 (3.4-ounce) box instant vanilla pudding mix
- 1 (12-ounce) container frozen whipped topping

Mix the pineapple(undrained) and instant pudding. Fold in whipped topping. Frost cake.

Jenelle Carroll
Pitts Baptist Church
Harrisburg, NC

LEMON NUT CAKE

- 1 pound margarine
- 2 cups sugar
- 3 cups plain flour
- 6 eggs
- 1 teaspoon baking powder
- 2½ cups white raisins
- 4 tablespoons lemon extract
- 3¼ cups chopped pecans

Cream margarine and sugar; beat in eggs. Coat raisins and nuts with some flour. Mix baking powder with remaining flour and add to first mixture, mixing well. Bake in greased tube pan at 325° for 1 hour and 30 minutes.

Neola Cleveland
First Baptist Church
Booneville, MS

FRESH PEAR CAKE

CAKE

- 1¼ cups cooking oil
- 2 cups sugar
- 2 eggs
- 3 cups plain or cake flour
- 1 teaspoon salt
- 1 teaspoon baking soda
- Spices of your choice
- 3 cups raw, chopped pears
- 1½ cups chopped nuts

Mix in order given and pour into 9 x 13 inch pan. Bake 1 hour at 325°. Cool in pan or cover with topping while still warm.

TOPPING

- 1 cup light brown sugar
- 1 stick margarine
- ¼ cup cream
- 1 teaspoon vanilla

Cook in small sauce pan 2 to 3 minutes, stirring constantly.

You can use apples rather than pears, if desired.

Juanita Collins
Crossroads Baptist Church
Valdosta, GA

OREO CAKE

- 1 (16-ounce) package Oreo Cookies
- 2 (3.4-ounce) packages instant pudding mix
- 3 cups milk
- 1 (8-ounce) package cream cheese
- 1 stick butter
- 1 (10-ounce) carton frozen whipped topping
- ½ cup powdered sugar

Crumble ½ package cookies into 9 x 13 inch glass dish. Mix pudding with 3 cups milk and beat until thick. Set aside. Mix cream cheese, butter and powdered sugar and fold in whipped topping. Mix with pudding and put on top of cookies. Crumble rest of cookies and put on top of pudding mix and refrigerate.

Jean Evans
Central Baptist Church Bearden
Knoxville, TN

HAWAIIAN SUNSET CAKE

CAKE

- 4 eggs
- ½ cup oil
- 1¼ cups sweet milk
- 1 (3.4-ounce) package instant vanilla pudding mix
- 1 (3-ounce) package orange Jell-O
- 1 (1 pound, 2-ounce) orange supreme cake mix

Mix all ingredients together. Beat until smooth. Pour into 3 greased and floured 9-inch cake pans. Bake at 350° for approximately 35 to 30 minutes. Cool well.

FILLING

Before starting cake, mix well and chill:

- 1 (20-ounce) can crushed pineapple, drained well
- 2 cups sugar
- 1 (8-ounce) package sour cream
- 1 (12-ounce) package frozen coconut, thawed

Remove 1 cup of filling for the topping. Split layers of cake and stack with the balance of the filling mixture.

TOPPING

- 1 cup filling
- 1½ cups frozen whipped frosting

Blend well. Spread on top and sides of cake. Place in air tight container and refrigerate.

Bobby Sue Green
Trinity Baptist Church
Childersburg, AL

EARTHQUAKE CAKE

- 1 cup chopped pecans
- 1 cup coconut
- 1 (1 pound, 2-ounce) box German Chocolate cake mix
- 1 (8-ounce) package cream cheese
- 1 stick margarine
- 1 (16-ounce) box powdered sugar

Grease 9 x 13 inch pan. Spread pecans and coconut on bottom of pan. Mix cake as directed on box. Pour over pecans and coconut. Melt cream cheese and margarine and add powdered sugar. Pour over cake and bake in heated 350° oven for 1 hour or until brown.

Donnie Garrison
Twin Lakes Baptist
Walls, MS

COAL MINER'S CAKE

CAKE

- 1 (1 pound, 2-ounce) box devil's food cake mix
- 1 (16-ounce) can cherry pie filling
- 2 eggs
- 1 teaspoon vanilla

Beat eggs with a fork. Add cherries, cake mix and vanilla. Stir gently with a spoon until mixed (do not beat). Pour into a greased 9 x 13 inch pan and bake at 350° for 30 to 35 minutes. While cake bakes, prepare following:

TOPPING

- 1 cup white sugar
- 1 stick margarine
- 1 cup chopped pecans
- ½ cup evaporated milk
- 1 cup chocolate chips

Bring to a boil, margarine, sugar and milk, stirring often. Boil for 1 minute and remove from heat. Add chocolate chips. Stir until melted and add pecans; stir to mix. Pour over cake as soon as it is taken from oven.

Faye Swebster
Glencoe, KY

SCRIPTURE CAKE

1 cup Judges 5:25 last clause Cream
1 cup Jeremiah 6:20 Sugar
2 cups I Samuel 30:12
1 cup Numbers 17:8
1 cup Judges 4:19 (last clause) milk
2 cups Nahum 3:12 (optional)
2 tablespoons I Samuel 14:25
II Chronicles 9:9—season to taste
6 Jeremiah 17:11
4½ cups I Kings 4:22
2 tablespoons Amos 4:5
a pinch of Leviticus 2:13

Mix all ingredients well. Pour into tube or Bundt pan that has been well greased and floured. Bake at 350° for 1 hour and 30 minutes or until done when tested.

May God bless you as you bake.

Lucille Clark
Highland Baptist Church
Vicksburg, MS

FROSTING CAKE

CAKE

1 (1 pound, 2-ounce) package yellow cake mix
1 cup oil
1 cup water
4 eggs

Mix well and add:

½ cup nuts
1 can Coconut-Pecan Frosting Mix

Mix well. Pour into greased tube or loaf pan and bake at 325° for 45 to 55 minutes until tests done. Let cool and ice with

1 can Sour Cream Frosting Mix

You can use different cake mixes and different frostings to make these cakes.

Maxine Boyette
Keatchie, LA

CHOP SUEY CAKE

CAKE

- 2 cups plain flour
- 2 cups sugar
- 2 eggs
- 1 (20-ounce) can crushed pineapple, undrained
- 2 teaspoons soda
- ½ teaspoon salt
- 1 cup chopped nuts

Mix all ingredients well. Bake in 9 x 13 inch greased and floured pan until tests done. While cake is hot frost with:

FROSTING

- 1 (8-ounce) package cream cheese
- 1 stick margarine
- 2 cups powdered sugar
- 1 teaspoon vanilla
- 1 cup chopped nuts

Mix well spread on warm cake.

Joyce Hudson

PUMPKIN PIE CAKE

- 3 eggs
- ½ cup brown sugar
- ½ cup white sugar
- 2 teaspoons vanilla
- ½ teaspoon salt
- 1 (1 pound, 2-ounce) box butter cake mix
- 1 (14-ounce) can pumpkin
- 1 (12-ounce) can condensed milk
- 2 cups pecans
- 1 stick margarine

Combine eggs and brown and white sugars. Add pumpkin, condensed milk, vanilla and salt to egg mixture. Pour into greased 9 x 13 inch pan. Sprinkle cake mix over the pumpkin mixture and press slightly. Sprinkle pecans over this mixture. Melt 1 stick margarine and spoon over pecans. Bake 350° (325° for glass) for 50 minutes.

Alice Benson

YUM-YUM CAKE

CAKE
2 cups self-rising flour
2 eggs
2 cups sugar
1 (20-ounce) can crushed pineapple with juice

Mix all together. Pour in greased 9 x 13 pan. Bake 325° for 35 to 45 minutes. Cake will look white and not done.

TOPPING
1 (5-ounce) can evaporated milk
1 cup sugar
1 cup chopped pecans
1 cup coconut
1 stick margarine

Mix all together. Cook over low heat until boiling. Pour over hot cake.

Margaret Boutwell
First Baptist Church
Bay Minette, AL

TROPICAL FANTASY

1 (1 pound, 2-ounce) box yellow cake mix
3 medium to large eggs
¾ cup oil
1 (11-ounce) can mandarin oranges with juice

Combine cake mix, eggs, oil and oranges with juice in large mixing bowl. Mix according to directions on cake mix box. Spray 9 x 13 inch pan with Pam. Pour mixture into pan. Bake at 350° for 30 to 35 minutes. Cool completely.

1 (20-ounce) can crushed pineapple with juice
1 (3½-ounce) can coconut
1 (3.4-ounce) box banana instant pudding
1 (10-ounce) carton frozen whipped topping, thawed

In medium bowl combine pineapple, coconut and pudding mix. Mix well and fold in thawed whipped topping. Spread on cooled cake.

Judy David
Northside Baptist Church
Lafayette, LA

CAJUN CAKE

2 sticks margarine
4 eggs
1½ cups all-purpose flour
2 cups sugar
½ cup cocoa
1 cup coconut
1 cup black walnuts, finely chopped
1 jar marshmallow creme
Vanilla or chocolate frosting mix

Mix all ingredients except marshmallow creme in large bowl. Pour into well greased and floured 9x13 inch pan. Bake in 350° oven for 20 to 25 minutes. Remove from oven and spread with marshmallow creme. Let cool and ice with favorite vanilla or chocolate frosting.

Dorothy Kelly
First Baptist Church
Ozark, MO

LEMON LOVER'S CAKE

1 (1 pound, 2-ounce) box lemon cake mix
1 (5-ounce) can frozen lemonade
1 cup sugar

Mix cake by directions. Bake in 9 x 13 inch pan. While cake is baking, melt on low heat (or in microwave) lemonade with 1 cup sugar. Pour over hot cake. Prick holes for a more strong juicy lemon flavor. No other frosting needed.

Great served with cheese slices or Cool Whip

Mary Jackie Callahan
Wayside Baptist Church
Miami, FL

ORANGE SLICE CAKE

CAKE

- 2 sticks margarine
- 2 cups sugar
- 4 eggs
- 3½ cups unsifted flour
- ½ cup buttermilk
- 1 teaspoon soda
- 1 (10-ounce) box dates, chopped
- 1 (3½-ounce) can coconut
- 1 (16-ounce) package orange slice candy, cut fine
- 2 cups chopped pecans
- 2 cups powdered sugar
- 1 cup orange juice

Add soda to buttermilk. Put ½ cup flour over dates, nuts, coconut and candy. Mix margarine, sugar and add eggs. Beat well; add milk then add to the 3 cups flour. Fold in nut mixture. Bake in greased 9 x 13 inch pan for 2½ hours at 350°.Mix powdered sugar and orange juice and pour over cake and let set 24 hours before cutting.

Freeze if you desire.

Hassie Taylor
Parkway Baptist Church
Orlando, FL

BUTTERFINGER CAKE

- 1 (1 pound, 2-ounce) box devil's food cake mix
- 1 (14-ounce) can sweetened condensed milk
- 1 (12-ounce) jar caramel ice cream topping
- 1 (12-ounce) container frozen whipped topping
- 2 king size Butterfinger candy bars

Mix cake mix as directed on box. Bake in 9 x 13 inch pan and turn out onto big flat piece of cardboard. With a straw, poke as many holes as you can in cake. Pour condensed milk all over cake, then pour caramel topping over cake. Then spread whipped topping which has been thawed over cake. Break up candy bars and sprinkle over top.

Jean Leonard
Indian Lake Baptist Church
Northport, AL

BLACK WALNUT CAKE

- 1 cup finely chopped black walnuts
- 3 eggs
- 2 cups all-purpose flour
- ⅔ cup milk
- ½ teaspoon salt
- 2 cups brown sugar
- 3 teaspoons baking powder
- ½ cup butter
- 1 teaspoon vanilla

Grease and flour 9 x 13 inch pan. Cream butter and sugar; add egg yolks and nut meats. Add sifted dry ingredients alternately with milk. Add vanilla. Beat egg whites until stiff and fold into cake mixture. Bake in 350° oven for 1 hour.

Louise Harrison
Ripley, MS

TURTLE CAKE

CAKE

- 1 (1 pound, 2-ounce) package Devil's Food Cake mix
- 1 (12-ounce) bag caramels
- ½ cup evaporated milk
- ½ cup chopped pecans

Mix cake according to directions on package. Pour ½ mixture into greased and floured 9 x 13 inch pan and bake 15 minutes at 375°. Heat caramels and milk in microwave until caramels are melted. Pour over cake being careful not to get to sides. Add pecans on top of caramel mixture. Top with remaining cake mix. Bake for 25 minutes. When cool, cover with following icing:

ICING

- 1 pound powdered sugar
- 2 tablespoons margarine
- 1 teaspoon vanilla
- Cocoa, as desired

Mix melted butter, powdered sugar, vanilla and enough cocoa to make icing as dark as desired. Spread over cake.

Margaret Caraway
First Baptist Church
Greensburg, LA

KENTUCKY WILDCAT CAKE

CAKE

- 2 cups flour
- 2 cups sugar
- 2 eggs
- 1 teaspoon vanilla
- 1 cup chopped walnuts
- 2 teaspoons baking soda
- 1 (20-ounce) can crushed pineapple, undrained

Mix all ingredients together and beat for 2 minutes at low speed. Bake at 350° in Bundt pan for 45 minutes. Let cook and remove from pan.

ICING

- 1 (8-ounce) package cream cheese
- ¼ cup margarine
- 1 teaspoon vanilla
- 1½ cups powdered sugar
- ¾ cup chopped pecans

Mix together and spread over cake.

Margie Hallett
1st Evangelical Methodist Church
Latonia, KY

PAYDAY CANDY BAR CAKE

- 1 (1 pound, 2-ounce) yellow cake mix
- 1 egg
- 2 sticks margarine
- ⅔ cups white corn syrup
- 1 (12-ounce) bag mini-marshmallows
- 1 (12-ounce) package peanut butter chips
- 2 cups dry roasted peanuts
- 2 cups crispy rice cereal

Mix cake mix, eggs and 1 stick margarine until crumbly. Put into 9 x 13 inch glass pan. Bake at 350° for 10 minutes. In a pan over low heat until melted, mix syrup, 1 stick margarine and peanut butter chips. Add peanuts and cereal. Mix together. Take cake out of oven and put marshmallows and then hot peanut mixture. Let cool (can even be put in refrigerator) and cut into squares.

Emma York
Prattmont Baptist Church
Prattville, AL

BOIL AND SPICE CAKE

CAKE

2 cups sugar
2 sticks margarine
2 cups warm water
2 teaspoons cinnamon
2 teaspoons nutmeg
2 teaspoons cloves
2 cups raisins

Place in saucepan and bring all to boil. Boil 2 minutes. Set off stove to cool. Sift together:

3 cups all-purpose flour
2 teaspoons soda
½ teaspoon salt
2 cups chopped pecans

When boiled mixture is completely cool, add the flour mixture and pecans. Stir just until mixed. Pour into a tube pan. Cook for 1 hour at 350°.

This can be frozen. It keeps well. If making for company or holidays the following frosting can be used:

FROSTING

2 cups powdered sugar
2 tablespoons margarine
3-4 tablespoons cold coffee
2 tablespoons cocoa
½ teaspoon vanilla

Cream butter, sugar and cocoa, add cold coffee (until thin enough to spread on cake) and ½ teaspoon vanilla. Frost cake and enjoy.

Loreva Sparks
New Chapel Hill Baptist
Calhoun, LA

GINGERBREAD CAKE

CAKE

- ½ teaspoon cinnamon
- ¼ teaspoon nutmeg
- ⅓ cup sugar
- 2 teaspoons baking powder
- ¼ teaspoon cloves
- 1½ cups plain flour
- 1 teaspoon ginger
- ¼ teaspoon salt
- ¼ cup butter
- ½ cup boiling water
- ½ cup molasses

Stir dry ingredients with whisk to blend. Combine butter and water. When butter melts, add molasses. Stir liquid into the flour mixture and mix with whisk just enough to make a smooth batter. Spread in shallow 8- or 9-inch square pan. Bake in 325° oven for 35 minutes. Serve hot with butter for breakfast or with applesauce or iced for dessert.

BUTTER FROSTING

- ¼ cup unsalted butter
- 1 egg yolk
- 1 cup powdered sugar
- 1 teaspoon vanilla

Beat butter until creamy. Stir in 1 egg yolk. Beat in powdered sugar (2 tablespoons at a time). Beat hard until light and fluffy. Flavor with vanilla and beat. Frost cake.

Maraget Bowne
St. Luke United Methodist Church
Pensacola, FL

MUSCADINE DUMP CAKE

2 cups fresh muscadine hulls
1½ cups pulp
1 cup sugar
1½ tablespoons lemon juice
2 tablespoons flour
⅛ teaspoon salt
¼ teaspoon cinnamon
1 (1 pound, 2-ounce) yellow cake mix
2 sticks margarine, melted
1 cup chopped pecans

Cook muscadine hulls and next 6 ingredients until slightly thickened. Pour into an 8 x 10 inch sheet cake pan. Sprinkle with dry cake mix. Spoon melted margarine over this and sprinkle with pecans. Bake for 1 hour at 325°.

Clovis Lee Hall
Providence Baptist Church
Shreveport, LA

EZEE DUMP CAKE

1 (20-ounce) can crushed pineapple with juice
1 (20-ounce) can cherry pie filling
1 (1 pound, 2-ounce) yellow cake mix
¾ cup melted margarine
½ cup flaked coconut
1 cup chopped pecans

Dump undrained pineapple and pie filling in 9 x 13 inch pan. Sprinkle cake mix over fruit. Drizzle melted butter. Add coconut and pecans. Bake 1 hour at 350°.

Serve warm or cold. Great when served with whi
ice cream.

Wh

LEMON LAYER DESSERT

- 1 stick butter
- 1 cup flour
- ½ cup crushed pecans
- 2 (3.4-ounce) boxes lemon instant pudding
- 3 cups milk
- 8 ounces cream cheese
- 1 (10-ounce) package Cool Whip
- ½ teaspoon vanilla

Melt butter in 9 x 13 inch dish. Add flour and press out to cover bottom. Sprinkle pecans on top. Bake at 350° for 15 to 20 minutes until light brown. Cool. Mix lemon pudding mix with milk and spread on top of crust. Mix cream cheese, 8 ounces of Cool Whip and vanilla and spread on top of pudding. Cool. Spread remaining Cool Whip on top before serving.

Wanda Henson
Parksville Baptist Church
Parksville, KY

GRANNY KEENUM'S CHOCOLATE PUDDING

- 2 egg yolks
- 1½ cups milk
- 3 tablespoons flour
- 3-4 tablespoons cocoa
- ½ stick butter
- 1 tablespoon vanilla flavoring
- 4 tablespoons sugar
- 2 egg whites

Mix egg yolks, sugar, milk, flour, cocoa, butter and vanilla flavoring. Cook on medium heat until thick, stirring frequently. Pour into oven-proof dish. Beat egg whites until stiff and add sugar. Cover pudding with topping and brown in 350° oven.

6 servings

Alyine Keenum
Enon Baptist Church
Trinity, AL

PERSIMMON PUDDING

1 cup persimmon pulp
1 cup sugar
1 cup flour
1 egg
½ stick butter
¼ teaspoon vanilla
1 cup milk

Mix well and bake 350° for 30 minutes or until done.

W. P Millsaps
Statesville, NC

PEANUT BUTTER BAR

1 large package Oreo cookies
1 stick margarine
½ gallon vanilla ice cream
⅔ cup chocolate chips
3 tablespoons margarine
2 cups powdered sugar
1 (12-ounce) evaporated milk
1 teaspoon vanilla
1 package Spanish peanuts
Chocolate sauce

Crush Oreo cookies and mix in bowl with stick of melted margarine. Press lightly into 9 x 13 inch glass dish. Freeze for one hour. Set out ½ gallon ice cream to soften. Then spread over frozen crust and refreeze. Melt chocolate chips and 3 tablespoons margarine together. Add powdered sugar, evaporated milk and vanilla and mix. Boil mixture 8 to 10 minutes. Let cool completely. Sprinkle peanuts over ice cream. Pour chocolate sauce over all this. Freeze overnight before serving. Keep leftovers frozen.

Carolyn Maddox
Holly Grove Baptist Church
Brownsville, TN

PEACH COBBLER

½ cup butter
1 (16-ounce) can sliced peaches
1¼ cups sugar, divided
1 cup milk
2 teaspoons baking powder
¼ teaspoon salt

Melt butter in 2-quart baking dish; set aside. Drain peaches, reserving ¼ cup juice. In a saucepan, bring the peaches and fruit just to a boil. Meanwhile in a mixing bowl, combine 1 cup sugar, flour, milk, baking powder and salt, mixing well. Pour over butter in baking dish. Spoon hot peaches over batter. Sprinkle with remaining sugar. Bake at 400° for 25 minutes or until cake tests done. Serve warm.

6-8 servings

Betty Jones
Dothan, AL

BEST EVER APPLE COBBLER

½ cup butter
2 cups sugar
2 cups water
1½ cups sifted self-rising flour
½ cup shortening
⅓ cup milk
2 cups finely chopped apples
1 teaspoon cinnamon

Melt butter in a 9 x 13 inch baking dish. Heat sugar and water together. Meanwhile cut shortening into flour until like fine crumbs. Add milk and stir with a fork until dough leaves the side of bowl. Turn out on floured board; knead until smooth. Roll dough into a large rectangle about ¼ inch thick. Sprinkle cinnamon over apples and spread over dough evenly. Roll up like a jelly roll. Slice in about ½-inch pieces. Place in pan with melted butter. Pour sugar syrup carefully over rolls. (This looks like too much liquid but the crust absorbs it) Bake at 350° for 55 to 60 minutes.

This cobbler maybe made with other fresh, frozen or canned fruits, such as blackberries, blueberries, cherries, peaches or strawberries. If packed in liquid, drain and substitute for part of the sugar syrup. Always use 2 cups of liquid.

Jane Williamson
First Baptist Church
Estill Springs, TN

CHOCOLATE DELIGHT

- ¾ cup butter, melted
- 1½ cups flour
- ¾ cup chopped pecans
- 1 (8-ounce) package cream cheese, softened
- 1 cup powdered sugar
- 1 (12-ounce) carton frozen whipped topping, divided
- 1 (3.4-ounce) instant vanilla pudding
- 1 (4.6-ounce) instant chocolate pudding
- 3 cups milk
- 1 cup chopped pecans
- Grated chocolate

Combine butter, flour and pecans, mixing well. Press into 13 x 9 inch dish. Bake at 375° for 15 minutes. Cool completely. Combine cream cheese, powdered sugar and 1½ cup whipped topping; blend thoroughly. Spread over crust and cool. Combine pudding mixes and milk, beat 2 minutes at medium speed. Spread over cream cheese layer. Spread remaining whipped topping over pudding layer. Garnish with pecans and chocolate. Refrigerate.

15 servings

Delores Garris
Mt. Beulah Baptist Church
Wadesboro, NC

CHOCOLATE LAYER DESSERT

- 1 cup self-rising flour
- 1 cup chopped pecans
- 1 stick melted margarine
- 1 (8-ounce) package cream cheese
- 1 cup powdered sugar
- 1 cup frozen topping
- 2 (3.4-ounce) instant chocolate pudding mixes
- 3 cups milk
- 1 (10-ounce) carton frozen topping

Mix flour, pecans and margarine. Press in 9 x 13 inch pan. Cook at 350° for 10 to 12 minutes. Cool completely. Blend cream cheese, sugar and 1 cup frozen topping. Spread evenly over crust. Mix pudding and milk. Spread evenly. Top with frozen topping and sprinkle with nuts. Keep refrigerated.

Eleanor Kay
Whitesburg Baptist Church
Huntsville, AL

BUTTERSCOTCH SPECIAL

- 1 stick margarine
- 1 cup plain flour
- 1 cup nuts, chopped
- 1 cup powdered sugar
- 1 (8-ounce) package cream cheese
- 1 (10-ounce) carton whipped topping
- 2 (3.4-ounce) packages butterscotch instant pudding
- 3 cups milk
- 1 (12-ounce) carton whipped topping

Mix softened margarine, flour and nuts; press in 9 x 13 inch pan and bake at 375° for 15 minutes. Mix powdered sugar, cream cheese and small frozen topping and press on top of crust. Then mix pudding mixes and milk and pour over top of other mixture. Top with large frozen topping.

Viola Brown
Holly Grove Baptist Church
Bells, TN

RICE PUDDING

- 2 quarts water
- ½ cup rice
- 2 cups sugar
- 1 teaspoon vanilla flavoring
- ½ stick butter
- 1½ cups milk
- 1 egg
- 1 teaspoon salt
- 3 tablespoons flour

Mix egg, salt, vanilla, sugar, milk and flour together and set aside. In a 3-quart saucepan, bring water to boil. When water boils, add rice. Reduce heat to a simmer; simmer for 45 minutes. Mixture must cook very slowly. When done, rinse with very hot water; return to stove and add butter. Let butter melt, then stir. Now add set aside mixture; place on low heat and stir mixture continuously until it thickens. Serve hot.

You can top your pudding with butter and evaporated milk after the pudding is placed in serving bowls.

Joyce Lamb
Crosspointe Baptist Church
Owensboro, KY

SOUTHERN BANANA PUDDING

1 (12-ounce) package vanilla wafers (may need more)
6 large bananas
1 (5.1-ounce) package instant vanilla pudding
1 (8-ounce) package sour cream
1 (10-ounce) carton frozen topping
2½ cups milk

Add milk and sour cream to vanilla pudding mix, mixing well. Layer wafers and bananas in dish. Add pudding mix. Top with frozen topping and vanilla wafer crumbs.

Verla Newman
Dania Beach, FL

RASPBERRY CHEESECAKE COOKIE PIZZA

¾ cup butter
¾ cup sugar
1 egg yolk
1 teaspoon vanilla
1½ cups all-purpose flour
1 (8-ounce) package cream cheese
1 egg
1 tablespoon sugar
⅓ cup seedless raspberry preserves
¼ cup sliced almonds, toasted

Beat butter with electric mixer on medium to high speed for 30 seconds. Add ¾ cup sugar and beat until combined. Beat in egg yolk and vanilla. Beat in as much of the flour as you can with mixer. Stir in remaining flour with wooden spoon. Spread dough in a lightly greased 12- or 13-inch pizza pan. Bake in a 350° oven for 25 minutes until golden brown. Meanwhile, beat together cream cheese, egg and 1 tablespoon sugar until smooth. Spread over hot crust to within ½ inch of edge. With a knife, carefully swirl preserves to marble. Sprinkle with almonds. Bake 5 to 10 minutes more until filling is set. Cook in pan on wire rack. Cut in wedges. Store in refrigerator.

12-16 servings

Wanda Jones
Montevallo, AL

EASY CHERRY PIE

1 (16-ounce) can sweetened cherry pie filling
1 (9-ounce) box Jiffy brand yellow cake mix
⅓ cup sugar
1 stick margarine, melted

Mix pie filling and sugar together. Pour into a greased 9-inch pie plate. Evenly sprinkle cake mix over cherry mixture. Make a small well in center of pie to prevent the pie from bubbling over. Pour melted margarine over cake mix. Bake at 350° until golden brown and bubbly.

Robert Mae Long
New Hope Baptist Church
Berry, AL

SUGARLESS APPLE PIE

8 medium apples
1 teaspoon cinnamon
½ teaspoon nutmeg
2 tablespoons butter
1 (12-ounce) can frozen apple juice concentrate
2 tablespoons cornstarch
2 (9-inch) deep dish pie shells (use 1 for topping)

Peel, core and slice apples. Put apples in unbaked pie shell. Melt apple juice; add spices, butter and cornstarch. Stir until thickened. Pour over apples. Put a top crust over apple mixture. Bake at 350° for 45 minutes or until done.

Mary Welch
Rosenberg, TX

DIABETIC MILLIONAIRE PIE

- ½ pint whipping cream, whipped
- 1 (15¼-ounce) can crushed pineapple, drained
- 9 packages sweet and low
- 1 box D-Zerta topping mix (2 packages)
- Juice of 3 lemons
- Graham cracker crust

Mix all the ingredients and pour into graham cracker crust; chill and serve.

Susie Hayes
Holly Grove Baptist Church
Bells, TN

OATMEAL PIE

- ⅔ cup sugar
- 1 stick margarine
- 2 eggs, beaten
- ⅔ cup white corn syrup
- ⅔ cup 1-minute oats
- 1 teaspoon vanilla
- 1 (9-inch) pie crust

Cream sugar and margarine. Blend in the two eggs. Add remaining ingredients and mix well. Pour into pie shell and bake at 365° for 55 to 60 minutes until done.

Robert Brown
Monticello, KY

MILLIONAIRE PIE

- 1 (20-ounce) can crushed pineapple, drained well
- 1 (14-ounce) can sweetened condensed milk
- ¼ cup lemon juice
- 1 (10-ounce) carton frozen whipped topping
- 1 cup chopped pecans
- 1 cup shredded coconut (optional)
- 2 graham cracker pie crusts

Mix condensed milk and lemon juice, then add drained pineapple and mix well. Add pecans and whipped topping. Beat well. Pour into pie crusts and chill until ready to use.

Can keep up to 1 year in freezer.

Lallage Seale
Pleasant Ridge Baptist Church
Hueytown, AL

IMPOSSIBLE SWEET POTATO PIE

- ¾ cup sugar
- ½ cup self-rising flour
- 2 tablespoons margarine
- 1 (12-ounce) can evaporated milk
- 2 eggs
- 2 cups cooked sweet potatoes
- 2½ teaspoons cinnamon
- 2 teaspoons vanilla

Heat oven to 350°. Grease pie plate. Beat all ingredients until smooth using blender or hand mixer. Pour into pie plate. Bake 50 to 55 minutes or until knife inserted in center comes out clean.

Betty Britt
Hyde Park Baptist Church
Lumberton, NC

CARAMEL PIE

4 (14-ounce) cans sweetened condensed milk
2 graham cracker crusts
1 (12-ounce) carton frozen whipped topping
Chocolate chips or pecans (optional)

Take paper off milk cans. Lay on sides in large boiler. Cover with water; boil 1½ to 2 hours, keeping the cans covered with water. Cool. Place contents of 2 cans in each pie shell and cool. Cover with whipped topping and sprinkle with chocolate chips or pecans.

Dapne Baldes
New Hope Baptist Church
Berry, AL

PUMPKIN PECAN PIE

1 (9-inch) pie shell
3 eggs
1½ cups pumpkin puree
¾ cup dark corn syrup
¾ cup white sugar
½ teaspoon ground cinnamon
¼ teaspoon salt
1 cup chopped pecans

Beat eggs until foamy; stir in pumpkin, corn syrup, sugar, cinnamon and salt. Pour into pie shell. Top with pecans. Bake at 350° for 50 to 60 minutes or until knife inserted in the center comes out clean.

Jeanette Davis
Jackson,

BUTTERMILK PIE

- 1 cup sugar
- 2 tablespoons flour
- ½ teaspoon salt
- 3 egg yolks
- 2 cups buttermilk
- 4 tablespoons butter
- 3 egg whites
- 1 (9-inch) pie shell

Combine sugar, flour and salt; beat lightly with egg yolks. Add buttermilk and butter, which has been mixed and cooled. Gradually add to dry ingredients and mix well. Thoroughly fold in stiffly beaten egg whites. Pour into unbaked pie shell and bake at 375° for 45 minutes.

Marcel Medling
Brevard, NC

LEMONADE PIE

- 1 small can frozen lemonade, thawed
- 1 (10-ounce) carton frozen whipped topping
- 1 (14-ounce) can sweetened condensed milk
- 1 graham cracker crust
- Lemon slices

Mix lemonade, whipped topping and milk. Pour into pie crust. Chill at least four hours or overnight. Garnish with lemon slices.

Gervis Jones
Woodlawn Baptist Church
Crestview, FL

BUTTERSCOTCH PIE

- ¼ cup cornstarch
- 1 cup brown sugar
- ¼ teaspoon salt
- 2 cups milk, scalded
- 2 egg yolks + 1 white
- 3 tablespoons margarine
- ½ teaspoon vanilla
- 1 (9-inch) pie crust, baked
- Whipped cream, if desired

In large microwave bowl mix cornstarch, brown sugar and salt, gradually adding scalded milk. Cook in microwave on high until mixture comes to boil and thickens. Stir occasionally. Remove dish from microwave and add small amount to beaten eggs. Stir into remaining mixture and cook 1 more minute. Add margarine and vanilla, mixing well. Cool slightly and pour into baked pie shell. Cool. Cover with whipped cream.

Donna Morrow
Fort Wayne, IN

PINTO BEAN PIE

- 1 cup cooked pinto beans with juice
- 1 (3½-ounce) can coconut
- 1 cup chopped nuts
- 4 whole eggs
- 3 cups sugar
- 1 tablespoon vanilla
- 2 sticks margarine
- 3 baked pie shells

Mash beans well. Beat eggs and add with other ingredients. Mix well. Pour into crusts and bake 45 to 60 minutes at 300°.

Ethel Styles
Locust Hill Baptist Church
Travelers Rest, SC

RHUBARB PIE

3 cups diced rhubarb
1 cup sugar
1 teaspoon grated orange peel
3 tablespoons flour
⅛ teaspoon salt
2 (9-inch) pie crusts (use 1 for top crust)
2 tablespoons butter

Mix all ingredients and put in pie shell. Top with butter and add top crust. Bake at 350° for 40 minutes.

Ava Peek
Merrimon Avenue Baptist Church
Asheville, NC

KENTUCKY STACK PIE

2 cups white sugar
2 cups brown sugar
2 sticks butter, melted
1 cup cream
6 tablespoons flour
2 teaspoons vanilla
6 whole eggs
5 pie shells

Remove flange from pie shells. Combine sugars and flour, add melted butter, cream, eggs and vanilla. Beat until smooth. Pour into unbaked pie crusts and bake in 300° oven for 30 minutes or until set. Remove from oven making sure filling is set in center and let cool 15 minutes. Leave one in pan. Remove other 4 pies from pans and stack on top. After completely cool this may be frosted with caramel ice cream icing if desired.

Make sure pies are set in center before letting them cool. This is a very rich pie so serve in small pieces. This recipe originated in Kentucky as a way of having enough to feed a number of people at family reunions or all day meetings..

Feeds approximately 30 people

Nancy B. Yocum
Hopewell Baptist Church
Harrodsburg, KY

CHESS PIE

- 3 eggs
- 1½ cups sugar
- 2 tablespoons cornmeal
- 1½ teaspoons vinegar
- 1 stick margarine
- 1 (9-inch) pie shell

Mix sugar and cornmeal together. Beat eggs, vinegar and melted margarine and mix with sugar and cornmeal. Pour into unbaked pie shell and bake at 325° for 45 to 60 minutes.

Ora Myers
Enon Baptist Church
Danville, AL

TRIP TO HAWAII PIE

- 1 (20-ounce) can crushed pineapple
- 1¼ cups sugar
- ¼ cup flour
- 1 (3-ounce) package orange gelatin
- 1 large can sour cherries, drained
- 1 cup chopped pecans
- 6 large bananas sliced
- 2 deep dish pie shells, baked
- Whipped topping, if desired

Cook crushed pineapple with liquid, sugar and flour until thickened. Add remaining ingredients and pour into baked pie shells. Chill and add whipped topping.

Keeps well in freezer

Linda Vaughn
Mt. Beulah Baptist Church
Morven, NC

JAPANESE FRUIT PIE

1 stick butter
1 cup sugar
2 eggs, beaten
1 tablespoon vinegar
Pinch of salt
½ cup pecans, chopped
½ cup frozen coconut
½ cup golden seedless raisins
1 (9-inch) pie shell

Mix sugar, butter, salt, eggs and vinegar. Add coconut, raisins and chopped pecans. Pour into unbaked pie shell and bake 35 to 40 minutes at 325° until golden brown.

Mable McCrory
Derma Baptist Church
Derma, MS

COCONUT PINEAPPLE PIE

1 cup sugar
3 tablespoons all-purpose flour
1 cup light corn syrup
1 cup flaked coconut
1 (8-ounce) can crushed pineapple with juice
3 eggs, beaten
1 teaspoon vanilla extract
1 unbaked 9-inch pastry shell
¼ cup butter, melted

In a bowl, combine sugar and flour. Add the syrup, coconut, pineapple, eggs and vanilla; mix well. Pour into pastry shell. Drizzle with melted butter. Bake at 350° for 50 to 55 minutes or until knife inserted near the center comes out clean. Cover loosely with foil if the top browns too quickly. Cool on a wire rack. Chill before cutting. Store in the refrigerator.

6-8 servings

Joyce Raulston
Hillside Baptist Church

PEANUT BUTTER PIE

- 1 chocolate crumb pie shell
- 1 (8-ounce) package cream cheese, softened
- 1 (8-ounce) carton frozen whipped topping
- 1 cup crunchy peanut butter

Mix peanut butter and cream cheese. Fold in whipped topping. Pour into crumb crust. Refrigerate.

Virginia Chambers

KENTUCKY PIE

- 1 (9-inch) pie shell
- 3 eggs, beaten
- 1 cup sugar
- 1 cup chocolate chips
- 1 cup chopped walnuts
- ½ cup self rising flour
- 1 teaspoon vanilla
- 1 stick butter, melted

Mix all ingredients together and put in a 9-inch pie shell. Bake 350° for 30 minutes. Let stand 20 minutes before cutting.

Edna Buff
Calvary Baptist Church
Morganton, NC

SOUTHERN PECAN PIE

- 1 cup white sugar
- 1 cup dark corn syrup
- 3 whole eggs, beaten
- 1 teaspoon vanilla
- 1 teaspoon vinegar
- 1 cup pecan halves.
- 1 (9-inch) pie shell

Combine all ingredients except pecans. Pour into unbaked pie shell and place pecan halves on top. Bake 1 hour at 350°.

Betty Isaacs
Porter Memorial
Lexington, KY

BROWN SUGAR PIE

- wn sugar, packed
- evaporated milk
- up water
- teaspoon salt
- 2 tablespoons cornstarch
- 1 teaspoon vanilla
- 2 eggs, slightly beaten
- 1 (9-inch) pie shell
- Frozen whipped topping for garnish

Mix all ingredients together and cook over medium heat until reaching bubbly boil stage. Pour in baked pie shell and cool. Serve with frozen whipped topping.

Peggy Lanham
Parksville Baptist Church
Parksville, KY

CLASSIC WALNUT PIE

- 3 eggs, lightly beaten
- 1 cup sugar
- 2 tablespoons all-purpose flour
- 1 cup corn syrup (dark or light)
- 2 tablespoons butter, melted
- 1 teaspoon vanilla
- 1 (9-inch) pastry shell
- 1½ cups large pieces walnuts

Heat oven to 400°. Combine eggs, sugar, flour, syrup, butter and vanilla. Blend well and pour into unbaked pie shell. Arrange walnuts on top. Bake in lower ⅓ of oven of 400° oven for 15 minutes. Reduce oven temperature to 350° and bake an additional 35 to 45 minutes or until center appears set. Cool completely.

8 servings

Patsy Smith
Amite, LA

REFRIGERATOR COOKIES

- 1 cup butter
- 2 cups sugar
- 2 eggs
- 3 cups flour
- 1 teaspoon soda
- ½ teaspoon salt
- 1 tablespoon vanilla
- 1 cup pecans (optional)

Cream butter, sugar and eggs. Then sift flour, soda, and salt together and add to butter and egg mixture. Add vanilla and pecans and shape into 2 or 3 rolls and chill overnight. Slice with sharp knife and bake 350° about 10 minutes.

These rolls freeze nicely to always have on hand.

Annice McCrory
Parkway Baptist Church
Kosciusko, MS

HEAVENLY COOKIES

- 1 cup margarine
- ½ cup powdered sugar
- 2 teaspoons vanilla
- 2 cups flour
- ½ cup nuts
- 1 cup quick cooking oats

Cream butter and sugar. Beat in vanilla. Add flour then nuts and oats. Shape into small balls. Bake at 325° for 25 to 30 minutes. While warm roll in powdered sugar.

Catherine Carter
Westwood Baptist Church
Alabaster, AL

OUTRAGEOUS COOKIES

- ½ cup butter
- ½ cup peanut butter
- 1 cup sugar
- 1 egg
- 1 teaspoon vanilla
- 1½ cups flour
- ½ cup oatmeal
- ½ teaspoon salt
- 1 teaspoon soda
- 1 (6-ounce) package chocolate chips
- ½ cup chopped nuts

Mix and roll into balls. Flatten with fork dipped in flour. Bake at 375° for 8 to 10 minutes.

Frances Neal
Providence Baptist Church
Shreveport, LA

CAN'T STOP COOKIES

- 2 cups sugar
- 2 cups butter
- 3 cups flour
- 2 teaspoons cream of tartar
- ½ teaspoon salt
- 2 teaspoons soda
- 4 cups cornflakes
- 1 cup chopped pecans

Cream sugar and butter. Add dry ingredients (sift flour, salt, soda, cream of tartar) Fold in nuts and cornflakes. Roll into quarter-size balls and bake at 350° for 10 to 15 minutes. They will be golden brown. Don't over bake.

Secret is real butter and not margarine.

Martha D. McNiel
Harlan Baptist Church
Harlan, KY

CHOCOLATE MACAROONS

2 egg whites
½ cup sugar
1 (6-ounce) package chocolate chips
1 teaspoon almond or vanilla extract
1 cup coconut

Whip egg whites stiff. Gradually add sugar. Add melted chocolate. Mix. Stir in coconut and flavoring. Drop on greased cookie sheet. Bake at 375° for 10 minutes.

Mozelle Wilson
Calvary Baptist Church
Morganton, NC

GERMAN CHOCOLATE COOKIES

1 box German chocolate cake mix
1 (5.1-ounce) box instant vanilla pudding
1 (12-ounce) bag milk chocolate chips
3 eggs
½ cup oil
1 cup chopped nuts

Stir all ingredients together. Bake at 350° for 10 to 12 minutes

You may have to add a few drops of water

Kattath Hornbuckle
Pleasant Garden Baptist Church

NOELS

- 2 teaspoons vanilla
- ½ cup powdered sugar
- 1 cup chopped nuts
- 1 cup margarine
- 2 cups flour

Cream together margarine and powdered sugar. Add remaining ingredients. Mix well. Shape into small balls and bake at 350° for 20 minutes. Partially cool and roll balls in more powdered sugar.

Sharon Stringfellow
New Hope Baptist
Tuscaloosa, AL

CEREAL COOKIES

- 2 cups Cheerios
- 2 cups graham cracker cereal
- 1 whole package of white almond bark, melted
- 1 (6-ounce) package peanuts

Mix together and spoon onto wax paper with a teaspoon.

Elaine Fuller
Westwood Baptist Church
Birmingham, AL

LONE RANGER COOKIES

- 2 cups butter
- 4 cups brown sugar
- 2 teaspoons vanilla
- 4 eggs, beaten
- 4 cups flour
- 1 teaspoon baking powder
- 2 teaspoons soda
- 2 teaspoons salt
- 2 cups quick cooking oatmeal
- 1 (12-ounce) package chocolate chips
- 4 cups crispy rice cereal

Cream together butter, brown sugar, vanilla and eggs and set aside. Mix together, flour, baking powder, soda, salt and remaining ingredients and fold into butter mixture.

Drop by spoon onto baking sheet. Bake at 350° for 10 to 12 minutes.

12 dozen

Myrtle S. Potter
Pensacola, FL

COCONUT COOKIES

- 1 cup butter
- 3 cups sugar
- 1 cup milk
- 40 large marshmallows
- 4 cups crushed graham crackers
- 3 cups coconut

Mix and boil butter, sugar and milk for 3 minutes. Remove from heat and add marshmallows. Let melt and add crushed graham crackers and coconut. Mix well. Drop on wax paper with teaspoon.

Approximately 50

Sarah Kerr
Holly Grove Baptist Church
Brownsville, TN

NO SUGAR COOKIE

- 2 cups all-purpose flour
- ½ cup butter
- ½ cup orange juice
- 1 teaspoon grated orange peel
- ½ teaspoon cinnamon
- ½ cup seedless raisins
- ½ cup walnuts, chopped
- 2 teaspoons baking powder
- 1 egg
- ½ teaspoon salt

In a large bowl with wooden spoon, stir all ingredients until well mixed; drop dough by tablespoon on greased cookie sheet 2 inches apart. Bake in a 375° oven for 20 minutes until lightly brown. Remove from cookie sheet. Store in tightly covered container.

2½ dozen

Betty Robertson
Troutman Baptist Church
Troutman, NC

MOLASSES COOKIES

- 1½ cups sugar
- ½ cup molasses
- 2 eggs, beaten
- 4 cups plain flour
- 2 teaspoons soda
- 2 teaspoons cinnamon
- 1 teaspoon cloves
- ½ teaspoon ginger
- sugar

Preheat over to 350°. Cream sugar and shortening. Sift all dry ingredients together. Add alternately the molasses, eggs and dry ingredients to the creamed mixture. Roll in 1-inch balls and roll in granulated sugar. Do not flatten. Place 2 inches apart on cookie sheet and bake until light brown. Do not overcook.

Trillie Brown
Chapel Hill Baptist Church
Northport, AL

OLD FASHIONED TEACAKES

1 cup sugar
½ cup butter
2 tablespoons buttermilk
1 egg
1 teaspoon vanilla
flour

Cream butter and sugar well. Add milk, egg, vanilla and enough flour to make batter thick. Roll batter thin and cut with cookie cutter. Bake at 350° 10 to 12 minutes until done.

2 dozen

Alyine Keenum
Enon Baptist Church
Trinity, AL

PUMPKIN CHOCOLATE CHIP COOKIES

1½ cups sugar
½ cup margarine or butter, softened
1 egg
2½ cups plain flour
1 teaspoon baking powder
1 teaspoon baking soda
1 teaspoon cinnamon
½ teaspoon salt
1 cup cooked or canned pumpkin
2 teaspoons vanilla
1 cup chocolate chips
1 cup chopped nuts

Cream sugar and butter with egg. Add dry ingredients and pumpkin. Stir in vanilla, chocolate chips and nuts. Drop by teaspoon on greased cookie sheet. Bake at 350° for 10 to 12 minutes.

Mona Fields
First Baptist Church
Aledo

CHOCOLATE CHIP CAKE COOKIES

- 1 (1 pound, 2-ounce) package white cake mix
- ½ cup vegetable oil
- 2 tablespoons water
- 1 cup chocolate chips
- 2 eggs
- ½ cup nuts

Mix and drop from teaspoon onto ungreased cookie sheet. Bake at 325° for 10 to 12 minutes. Cool 1 minute, then remove to rack.

About 4 dozen

Ruby Bentley
Lincolnton Baptist Church
Lincolnton, GA

3 INGREDIENTS COOKIES

- 1 cup peanut butter (creamy or crunchy)
- 1 egg
- 1 cup sugar
- Chocolate kisses or Junior Mint patties (optional)

Mix together and drop by teaspoon on ungreased cookie sheet. Bake 8 to 10 minutes. When removed from the oven set a chocolate kiss or Junior Mint pattie on top or eat plain.

1 dozen small cookies

Shirley Cunningham
First Baptist Church
Estille Springs, TN

OVER NIGHT COOKIES

- 1 cup white sugar
- 1 cup brown sugar
- 1 cup shortening
- 3 eggs
- 1 teaspoon vanilla
- 2 cups plain flour
- 1 teaspoon soda
- Pinch of salt

Cream shortening and sugars well and beat in eggs and vanilla. Sift flour, soda and salt together. Work flour mixture into other ingredients. Take out and divide in 2 parts. Work in flour until sticky. Put in refrigerator overnight. Take out and roll in balls and bake at 350° for 10 to 15 minutes.

Mary Anne Springer
First Baptist Church
Loretto, TN

BOILED OATMEAL CHOCOLATE COOKIES

- 3 tablespoons cocoa
- 2 cups sugar
- ½ cup milk
- ¼ stick margarine
- 1 cup nuts
- 2½ cups quick-cooking rolled oats
- 2 teaspoons vanilla
- ½ cup peanut butter

Mix and cook first 4 ingredients to rolling boil, time and cook 1½ minutes. Remove from heat and add last 4 ingredients. Mix well and drop on waxed paper. Cool.

Yvonne Sherrill
Mt. Hebron Baptist Church
Spruce Pine, AL

ICE BOX OATMEAL COOKIES

- 1 (16-ounce) box light brown sugar
- 2 cups sugar
- 1 pound butter or margarine
- 3 cups plain unsifted flour
- 2 teaspoons soda
- 7 cups oatmeal
- 2 teaspoons vanilla
- 4 eggs
- 1 cup coconut or cherries or pecans (your choice)

Cream sugar and butter or margarine. Add eggs, beat well and add flour sifted with soda then remaining ingredients. Shape into rolls. May be kept frozen and used as needed. Slice, bake at 375° for 10 minutes.

Polly Miller
First Baptist Church
Mathiston, MS

HAYSTACKER COOKIES

- ½ cup white chocolate chips
- 2 cups flaked coconut
- ½ cup white sugar
- ⅓ cup all-purpose flour
- 2 eggs
- ¼ cup finely chopped almonds
- ½ teaspoon vanilla extract

Melt chocolate in double boiler, in a saucepan over low heat or in microwave, stirring occasionally until smooth. In a large bowl combine coconut, sugar, flour, eggs, almonds and vanilla. Stir well. Fold in melted chocolate. Drop by rounded spoonfuls onto baking sheets. Bake in 350° oven for 25 minutes until set.

2 dozen

Rita Godwin
East Booneville Baptist Church
Booneville, MS

GRANNY'S SUGAR COOKIES

- 1½ cups granulated sugar
- 1½ cups butter
- 4 cups flour
- 1 teaspoon vanilla
- 8 teaspoons milk
- 3 teaspoons baking powder
- ½ teaspoon salt
- 2 eggs

Cream butter and sugar. Sift baking powder, salt and flour together. Beat eggs, add vanilla and milk, then flour. Mix well. Roll into balls about size of eggs and flatten with a glass dipped in sugar. Bake 10 to 12 minutes in 350° oven.

I sometimes add ½ cup blanched slivered almonds and use 1 teaspoon of almond extract.

Kaye Pavlescak
Medina, OH

CHOCOLATE COCONUT PECAN COOKIES

- 2 sticks butter or margarine
- 2 cups sugar
- 2 eggs
- 2 tablespoons light corn syrup
- 2 teaspoons vanilla
- 2 cups flour
- ¾ cup unsweetened cocoa powder
- 1 teaspoon soda
- 1½ cups shredded or flaked coconut
- 1 cup chopped pecans

In large bowl beat butter and sugar with electric mixer on medium until light and fluffy (1 to 2 minutes). Add eggs, corn syrup and vanilla; beat until well blended. Beat flour, cocoa and baking soda until thoroughly mixed. Stir in coconut and pecans. Drop by heaping tablespoonful onto ungreased cookie sheet. Do not flatten cookies. Bake in 375° oven for 10 to 11 minutes Let cook 1 to 2 minutes on pans, then remove to racks to cool completely.

3½ dozen

Alice Rickman
Pinewood Baptist Church
Pinewood, SC

7 LAYER COOKIES

1 stick melted margarine
2 cups graham cracker crumbs
1 (12-ounce) package chocolate chips
1 (12-ounce) package butterscotch chips
1 cup nuts
1 (5-ounce) package frozen coconut
1 (14-ounce) can sweetened condensed milk

Mix margarine and graham cracker crumbs. Then add ingredients as listed. Bake at 325° for 30 minutes. Cool and cut into bars.

Carolyn Harrill
Liberty Baptist Church
Ellenboro, NC

POTATO CHIP COOKIES

3½ cups flour
1 cup sugar
1 pound margarine
1 cup crushed potato chips
2 teaspoons vanilla

Cream sugar and margarine. Add flour a little at a time. Add vanilla and chips. Drop from spoon onto cookie sheet. Bake at 350° for 12 minutes or until brown.

Lois Morris
Crosspointe Baptist Church
Owensboro, KY

EASY COOKIES

1 (1 pound, 2-ounce) box cake mix (any flavor)
½ cup oil
2 eggs, beaten

Mix above ingredients. Do not add any other liquid. If desired add raisins, nuts, dates, chocolate chips, etc. Place walnut-size balls of dough on lightly greased baking sheet. Flatten each cookie with palm. Bake 325° for 8 to 10 minutes until barely done. When cookies begin to rise, pop pan up and down on oven rack for a chewy cookie and be sure not to overbake, otherwise cookies will be crunch.

Billie Farris
Second Baptist Church
Kings Mountain, NC

SPECIAL K COOKIES

1 cup sifted flour
½ teaspoon soda
½ teaspoon salt
½ cup margarine
1 egg
⅔ cup sugar
1 teaspoon vanilla
3 cups Special K

You will need more than three cups cereal

Sift flour, soda and salt. Cream margarine, sugar, and vanilla. Add egg. Beat well. Stir in dry ingredients, add 1 cup Special K. Roll teaspoon of dough in remainder of Special K. Bake on ungreased cookie sheet at 350° about 10 minutes. Remove and cool.

Mary Greenwood
Fellowship Baptist Church
Walkertown, SC

CONGO SQUARES

- 2½ cups self-rising flour
- 3 eggs
- 1 (16-ounce) box brown sugar
- 1 stick margarine or butter
- 1 (6-ounce) package chocolate chips
- 1 cup nuts

Mix sugar and butter until creamy. Mix rest of ingredients and spread into pan. Bake 20 to 25 minutes at 350° in an 11 x 13 inch pan.

Edna Brooks
Holly Grove Baptist Church
Bells, TN

FUDGY TOFFEE BARS

- 1¾ cups all-purpose flour
- ¾ cup powdered sugar
- ¼ cup baking cocoa
- ¾ cup cold butter or margarine
- 1 (14-ounce) can sweetened condensed milk
- 1 teaspoon vanilla extract
- 2 cups semisweet chocolate chips, divided
- 1 cup coarsely chopped walnuts
- ½ cup flaked coconut
- ½ cup English toffee bits or almond brick

In a bowl, combine flour, sugar and cocoa. Cut in butter until mixture resembles coarse crumbs. Press firmly into a greased 13 x 9 x 2 inch baking pan. Bake at 350° for 10 minutes. In a saucepan, heat milk, vanilla and 1 cup of chocolate chips, stirring until smooth. Pour over the crust. Sprinkle with nuts, coconut, toffee bits and remaining chocolate chips; press down firmly. Bake for 18 to 20 minutes.

3 dozen

Mrs. David Grigsby
Subligna Baptist Church
LaFayette, GA

QUICK EASY BARS

42 soda crackers
1 cup butter
1 cup brown sugar
Chopped nuts

Line a 12 x 15 inch cookie sheet with foil. Grease foil with butter. Place a layer of crackers on foil. Sprinkle with nuts. In small saucepan mix butter and sugar. Place over medium heat and boil for 3 minutes, stirring constantly. Spoon over crackers and nuts. Bake at 400° for 5 minutes. Cool and cut into squares.

Jeanette Statom
Westlawn Baptist Church
Huntsville, AL

HONEY BARS

1 cup sugar
¾ cup oil
¼ cup honey
1 egg
2 cups flour
½ teaspoon cinnamon
1 cup chopped nuts

Mix all ingredients. Bake in 350° oven for about 25 minutes or until golden brown.

ICING FOR HONEY BARS

1 cup powdered sugar
1 teaspoon water
2 tablespoons mayonnaise
1 teaspoon vanilla

Mix together and spread on cake mixture while hot. Use regular size cookie sheet.

Edith Flippo
First Baptist Church
Loretto, TN

PECAN PIE BARS

- 2 cups all-purpose flour
- ½ cup sugar
- ⅛ teaspoon salt
- ¾ cup butter or margarine, cut up
- 1 cup firmly packed brown sugar
- 1 cup light corn syrup
- ½ cup butter or margarine
- 4 eggs, lightly beaten
- 2½ cups finely chopped pecans
- 1 teaspoon vanilla

Combine flour, sugar and salt in a large bowl; cut in ¾ cup of butter thoroughly with a pastry blender until mixture resembles very fine crumbs. Press mixture evenly into a 13 x 9 inch greased pan, using a piece of plastic wrap to press crumb mixture firmly into pan. Bake at 350° 17 to 20 minutes or until lightly brown. Combine brown sugar, corn syrup and ½ cup butter in a saucepan; bring to a boil over medium heat, stirring gently. Remove from heat. Stir ¼ of the hot mixture into beaten eggs; add eggs to remaining hot mixture. Stir in pecans and vanilla. Pour filling over crust. Bake at 350° for 35 minutes or until set. Cool completely in pan on a wire rack. Cut into bars.

16 large bars

Catherine Carter
Westwood Baptist Church
Alabaster, AL

SPICE BARS

¾ cup oil
¼ cup honey or syrup
1 cup sugar
1 egg
1 teaspoon vanilla
2 cups flour
1 teaspoon soda
1 teaspoon cinnamon

Mix oil, honey, sugar, egg and vanilla, blending well. Sift flour, soda and cinnamon together and gradually add to batter mix. Batter will be stiff. Pour into a greased and floured 9 x 13 inch pan. Bake 350° for 20 minutes.

GLAZE FOR SPICE BARS

½ cup powdered sugar
2 teaspoons water
1 rounded teaspoon Miracle Whip

Mix together like thick cream. Spread on warm cake.

Mary Whitlow
First Baptist Church
Queen City, TX

CHESS SQUARES

1 stick margarine
1 (1 pound, 2-ounce) box yellow cake mix
2 eggs, beaten

Mix well with fingers. Pour and spread in jelly-roll pan. Mash to sides with hands.

1 (8-ounce) package cream cheese
1 (16-ounce) package powdered sugar
1 egg, beaten

Mix and pour over crust above. Spread evenly. Bake at 325° 10 to 12 minutes until lightly browned. When totally cooled, cut in small bars.

Casteva Corley
First Baptist Church
Bay Minette, AL

BANANA-PECAN SQUARES

1½ cups flour
½ teaspoon baking soda
½ teaspoon salt
½ cup butter or margarine
¾ cup sugar
1 egg
1 teaspoon vanilla
1 cup mashed bananas
½ cup chopped pecans
9 pecan halves (optional)

Mix flour, baking soda, and salt and set aside. In medium bowl cream butter and sugar until light and fluffy. Beat in egg, vanilla and banana (mixture will look curdled). Stir in flour mixture until well blended. Stir in chopped pecans. Spread into 9-inch square pan that has been greased. (May place pecans across top where squares will be cut, if desired). Bake in preheated 350° oven 25 minutes or until brown. Cool in pan. Cut into squares.

Neola Cleveland
First Baptist Church
Booneville, MS

CHEWY BARS

2 cups self-rising flour
3 eggs
1 stick butter or margarine
1 tablespoon vanilla
1 box light brown sugar

Mix batter together, then add any or all of the following:

1 cup coconut
1 cup raisins or dates
1 cup chopped nuts

Bake at 300° for 40 minutes in a 9 x 13 inch pan that has been greased and floured.

Susan B. Fowler
Clear Spring Baptist Church
Simpsonville, SC

PUMPKIN BARS

4 eggs
1⅔ cups sugar
1 cup oil
1 (16-ounce) can pumpkin
2 cups plain flour
1 teaspoon soda
1 teaspoon salt
2 teaspoons cinnamon

Heat eggs, sugar, oil and pumpkin until light and fluffy. Sift together dry ingredients and stir into pumpkin mixture. Bake at 350° 25 to 30 minutes in a 10 x 15 x 1 inch pan.

8 ounces cream cheese
1 stick butter
2 cups powdered sugar
2 teaspoons vanilla

Mix together and spread on cooled cake. Cut into bars.

Patsy Smith
Amity, LA

NEVER FAIL FUDGE

1 (12-ounce) can evaporated milk
5 cups sugar
2 sticks margarine
1 (12-ounce) package semi-sweetened chocolate chips
4 squares unsweetened chocolate, chipped
1 pound package marshmallows
2 cups nuts, chopped

Melt butter in large saucepan. Add sugar and milk. Bring to a boil and boil six minutes, stirring constantly. Remove from burner. Add marshmallows, chocolate chips, chocolate squares and nuts. Stir until the chocolate and marshmallows are melted. Stir rapidly for one minute. Pour into large well-buttered 17½ x 12 inch pan. Cool and cut into squares.

5 pounds

Dorothy A. Watts
Bay Minette, AL

7 POUNDS OF FUDGE

4 (1 pound) boxes powdered sugar
1 cup cocoa
1 pound margarine
1 pound Velveeta cheese
1 cup chopped nuts
2 tablespoons vanilla

Sift sugar and cocoa together. In top of double boiler, melt cheese and margarine. When melted, pour over dry ingredients; mix well with wooden spoon. Stir in vanilla and nuts. Pour into 15 x 17 inch buttered pan. Refrigerate.

Freezes good — I usually divide into small foil pans and share with friends

Lib Hughes
Westview Baptist Church
Sheby, N.C.

VELVEETA FUDGE

1	pound margarine	1	pound Velveeta cheese
4	pounds powdered sugar	1	cup cocoa
1	teaspoon vanilla	1	cup chopped nuts

Melt margarine and cheese together until very hot. Pour over powered sugar and cocoa. Add vanilla and nuts. Stir until smooth. Pour onto greased cookie sheet. Chill and cut. Keep refrigerated.

Carolyn Mace
Amboy Baptist Church
North Little Rock, AR

EASY CHOCOLATE FUDGE

4½	cups sugar	4	small, plain chocolate bars
½	stick margarine	1	pint marshmallow creme
1	(12-ounce) can evaporated milk	2	teaspoons vanilla
2	(12-ounce) packages chocolate chips	2	cups nuts

Mix sugar, margarine and milk together, stirring constantly. Bring to strong boil and boil 8 minutes. May turn curdly, that's O.K. Remove from heat and add chocolate chips and chocolate bars immediately. Stir until dissolved. Add marshmallow creme, vanilla and nuts. Blend and turn into greased glass dishes.

You will need help to stir. No beating needed. You are ready to pour when all ingredients are blended

5 pounds

Dorothy Kelly
First Baptist Church
Ozark, MO.

JINGLE BELL FUDGE

1 (12-ounce) package butterscotch chips
½ cup chunky peanut butter
⅔ cup sweetened condensed milk
½ cup walnuts, chopped

Combine butterscotch chips and peanut butter in top of double boiler until butterscotch melts. Stir until blended; add milk and stir just until blended. Spread in a foil lined 8-inch square pan. Press chopped nuts into surface and chill until firm. Cut into 1-inch squares.

64 servings

Wanda Jones
Montevallo, AL

49'S BARS

2 cups biscuit mix
1 (16-ounce) box brown sugar
4 eggs
2 tablespoons vanilla
2 cups pecans

Mix well. Pour into greased 13 x 9 inch or smaller pan (for thicker bars). Bake at 350° for 30 minutes or until done.

Patricia Bunton
First Baptist Church
Windsor, SC

BABY RUTH BARS

1	cup white Karo syrup	1	cup sugar

Bring to a boil and add:

12	ounces chunky peanut butter	4	cups Rice Krispies

Press into a buttered 9 x 13 inch pan.

12	ounces chocolate chips	6	ounces butterscotch chips

Melt together and pour over Rice Krispies mixture. Chill about 30 minutes and cut into pieces. Does not have to be refrigerated.

Doris Graham
Pinewood Baptist Church
Pinewood, SC

DATE FINGERS

1	stick margarine	1	egg, beaten
1	cup granulated sugar	2½	cups Rice Krispies
1	cup chopped dates	1	teaspoon vanilla
½	cup chopped pecans		Coconut or pecans (optional)

Cook margarine, sugar, dates, pecans and egg for 10 minutes over low/medium heat, stirring constantly. Remove from heat and cool until can be handled. Add Rice Krispies and vanilla. Shape into desired shape (i.e. balls, fingers, etc) then roll in coconut and/or nuts. Store in covered tin with waxed paper between layers.

Frances M. Mabe
Robinhood Road Baptist Church
Winston-Salem, N.C.

DATE NUT CANDY

- ½ cup margarine
- 8 ounces chopped dates
- 1 cup sugar
- 1 teaspoon vanilla
- 2 cups Rice Krispies
- 2 cups chopped pecans
- 1 cup flaked coconut (I use more)

Mix margarine, dates, sugar and vanilla in large saucepan and cook over low heat 10 minutes, stirring constantly. Remove from heat; add Rice Krispies and pecans. Shape into 3 logs; roll in coconut. Put in refrigerator until ready to slice.

Mary Greenwood
Fellowship Baptist Church
Walkertown, S.C.

CHOCOLATE POPCORN

- 2 bags microwave popcorn
- 1 (16-ounce) package Sathers chocolate
- 2 tablespoons creamy peanut butter
- 3 cups Rice Krispies
- 2 cups unsalted peanuts

Pop popcorn; remove all kernels that did not pop. In microwave safe bowl, melt chocolate for 3 minutes. Turn bowl after each minute and stir. Add peanut butter and stir until blended. In large container mix popcorn, Rice Krispies and peanuts together. Pour chocolate mixture over all and stir and lift with large spoon until all is covered with chocolate. Spread popcorn mixture evenly onto 2 large cookie sheets and let cool. Then break into pieces and store in large container.

Marjorie Engelhardt
First Baptist Church
Rosenberg, TX

FIESTA POPCORN

3 bags microwave popcorn
1 package almond bark
3 cups peanuts or M&M's

Pop the corn in microwave. Melt almond bark in microwave for 90 seconds and pour over popped corn. Add peanuts or M&M's and stir. Drop onto waxed paper.

Jo Williams
First Baptist Church
Amite, LA

DIVINITY

1½ cups sugar
½ cup water
2 tablespoons Karo syrup

Bring to boil and cook until softball stage. Add:

1 jar marshmallow creme
1 teaspoon vanilla
1 cup nuts

Beat until it starts getting thick. Drop by spoonfuls onto foil or pour into buttered pan.

Quinieve Bilton
Mimosa Lane Baptist Church
Mesquite, TX

NEW ORLEANS PRALINES À LA MICROWAVE

1 pound brown sugar
1 cup whipping cream

Mix together in 4-quart glass bowl. Microwave on high 14 minutes. Remove and add:

2 tablespoons butter
1 quart pecans

Stir till begins to thicken. Drop by spoonfuls onto foil. Let set until firm.

Paula Barron
Philadelphia Baptist Church
Deville, LA

PRALINES

1½ cups sugar
½ cup brown sugar
3 tablespoons white Karo syrup
½ cup whipping cream
1 stick butter
1 teaspoon vanilla
4 large marshmallows
3 cups pecans
Pinch of salt

In saucepan, mix the sugars, syrup, salt and whipping cream. Cook over medium heat to soft ball stage. Add butter, vanilla and marshmallows and beat until it begins to harden. Add nuts and drop by teaspoons onto waxed paper. Cool.

Louise Brown
First Baptist Church
Booneville, MS

THREE MINUTES PEANUT CHOCOLATE CLUSTERS

1 cup semi-sweet chocolate chips
2 cups Reeses peanut butter chips
2 cups unsalted dry roasted peanuts

Mix chips well. Put in microwave on high. Cook for 1½ minutes. Stir well. Cook for 1½ minutes more. Stir until the color is uniform. Add the peanuts and stir again. Spoon clusters on wax paper. Let stand 30 minutes or until firm. These can be put in the freezer.

10 servings

Gayle David
Northside Baptist Church
Lafayette, LA

HEAVENLY HASH

1 (6-ounce) package dry strawberry Jell-O (or any flavor)
1 (15-ounce) can fruit cocktail

Mix in large bowl and put in refrigerator for 30 minutes, then add:

1 (8-ounce) can crushed pineapple
1 (8-ounce) carton sour cream
1 (12-ounce) carton Cool Whip

Mix and keep refrigerated.

You can always add bananas, pecans, apples or any kind of berries if you want.

Anita Newberry
Alvin, Texas

POLAR SNACKS

- 6 cups Crispix cereal
- 3 cups Cheerios
- 2 cups dry roasted peanuts
- 2 cups plain M & M's
- 2 cups Eagle pretzels (small ones)
- 2 (12-ounce) bags polar stars or white chocolate chip morsels
- 1 teaspoon vegetable oil

Mix the 2 bags polar stars or chip morsels with vegetable oil and melt in microwave on high (1 minute-30 seconds). Mix well with other ingredients. Pour on a brown grocery bag to set. When cool, break into pieces.

Emma G. York
Prattmont Baptist Church
Prattville, AL

TEACHER'S BRUNCH

- 1 (12-ounce) box Corn Chex
- 1 (12-ounce) box Rice Chex
- 1 (15½-ounce) bag pretzels
- 1 large can nuts (any kind)
- 2 cups plain M&M's
- 2 cups peanut M&M's
- 2 cups dehydrated fruit, cut up

Mix together and store in air tight container

Wanda Jones
Montevallo, AL

BUCKEYES

1 cup butter
2 pounds powdered sugar
1 teaspoon vanilla
2 cups peanut butter

Mix well and roll into small balls. Add:

1 (16-ounce) bag chocolate chips
1 block paraffin

Melt chocolate chips with small amount of paraffin, dip balls with toothpick and place on waxed paper to cool.

Lula Helms
Selma, AL

CHURCH WINDOW CANDY

1 (10½-ounce) bag colored miniature marshmallows
1 (12-ounce) bag chocolate chips
1 cup pecans
1 stick margarine
1 can coconut

Melt chocolate chips and margarine. Let cool. Add nuts and marshmallows. Shape into a log and roll in coconut. Refrigerate for several hours. Slice to serve.

Elaine Fuller
Westwood Baptist Church,
Birmingham, AL

RYSTALLIZED PEANUTS

uts ½ cup water

cup sugar

In large heavy boiler mix above ingredients and cook on medium heat until all mixture has stuck to the peanuts, but has not turned white. Quickly pour onto a buttered 10 x 15 inch cookie sheet and sprinkle with salt. Separate peanuts. Bake in 300° oven for 15 minutes. Stir and bake another 15 minutes.

Elaine Fuller
Westwood Baptist Church
Birmingham, AL

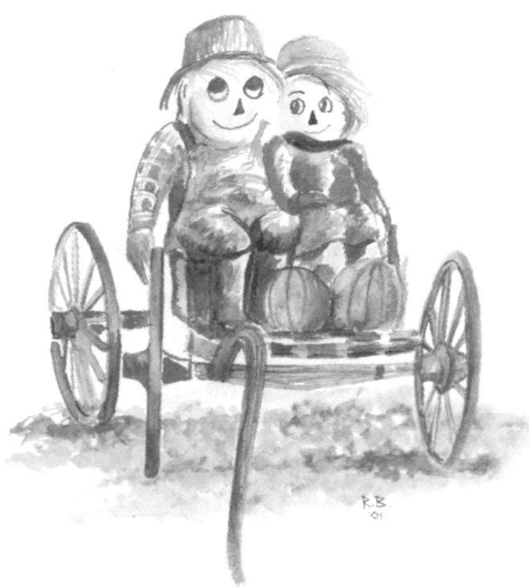

NO EGG HOMEMADE ICE CREAM

1 (5.1-ounce) box instant vanilla pudding mix
2 tablespoons cornstarch
1 quart half-and-half
1 cup sugar
2 tablespoons vanilla flavoring
½ gallon whole milk

You may substitute one 12-ounce can evaporated milk for half-and-half

Mix all ingredients. Pour into freezer and freeze as usual.

Clarice Thomas
Madison, AL

ICE CREAM SANDWICH DELIGHT

1 package ice cream sandwiches
2 large Butterfinger candy bars
1 (12-ounce) frozen whipped topping

Lay ice cream sandwiches close together in 9 x 13 inch dish. Top with Cool Whip. Repeat layering and after second topping of whipped topping, crumble Butterfinger bars and put on top. Freeze.

Delicious and Easy

Shirley Dike
Stetson Baptist Church
DeLand, FL

ORANGE SHERBET

1 (2-litre) orange soda
1 (20-ounce) can crushed pineapple
1 (14-ounce) can sweetened condensed milk

Mix together and put in ice cream freezer and freeze.

You must use orange soda and not orange juice.

Elizabeth Edwards
Pleasant Garden, NC

BUTTERFINGER ICE CREAM

1 jar marshmallow creme
1 (14-ounce) can sweetened condensed milk
6 Butterfinger candy bars
1 (8-ounce) carton frozen whipped topping
Whole milk

Beat creme and sweetened condensed milk. Crush Butterfingers and add to creme mixture, along with frozen whipped topping. Beat. Add whole milk to freeze line and freeze in ice cream freezer.

Edria Ann Norton
Sardis Springs Baptist Church
Athens, AL

CREAMY CHOCOLATE ICE CREAM

½ gallon chocolate milk (Nestles is best)
1 (12-ounce) carton frozen whipped topping
1 (14-ounce) can sweetened condensed milk

Mix well and freeze in ½ gallon container.

Very good and doesn't freeze real hard

Amy Beth Pressnell
Sardis Springs Baptist Church
Athens, AL

HOME-MADE ICE CREAM

1½ cups sugar
1 (5.1-ounce) instant vanilla pudding mix
1 (12-ounce) can evaporated milk
1 teaspoon vanilla flavoring
1 gallon milk

Mix real well and pour into freezer and finish filling with milk. Add fruit if you wish (peaches, strawberries, banana, etc.). Freeze as usual.

Rudy McCord
Bethel Baptist Church
Dothan, AL

PEANUT BUTTER ICE CREAM

- 1 (12-ounce) jar chunky peanut butter
- 1½ quarts half-and-half
- 6 large eggs
- 1 (14-ounce) can sweetened condensed milk
- 1 cup milk
- 1 tablespoon vanilla extract
- 2 cups sugar
- 2 tablespoons all-purpose flour

Cook peanut butter, 2 cups half-and-half and eggs in a Dutch oven over low heat, whisking constantly 7 minutes, or until a thermometer registers 160°. Whisk in remaining 4 cups half-and-half, condensed milk, milk and vanilla. Combine sugar and flour; whisk into hot mixture until sugar dissolves. Pour into 5-quart freezer and freeze.

Mrs. David Grigsby
Subligna Baptist Church
LaFayette, GA

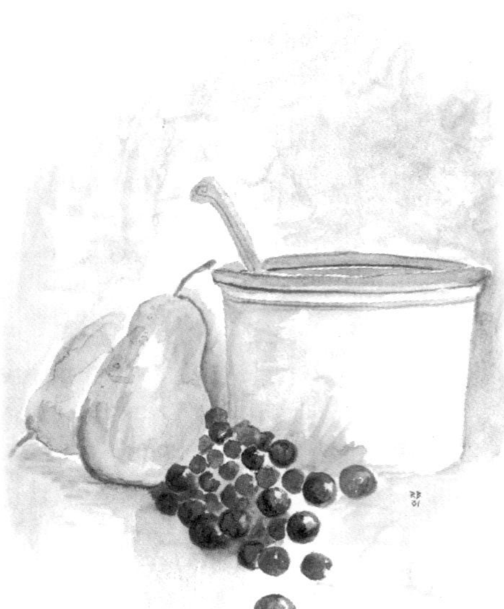

INDEX

C